Printed in USA

ISBN-978-1-7367197-6-3

Library Of Congress- 2021904930

DEDICATION

This book is dedicated to all of our loved ones who are no longer here with us and to everyone who was impacted by the Covid-19 pandemic. May this book bring you comfort knowing that we all went through this period together.

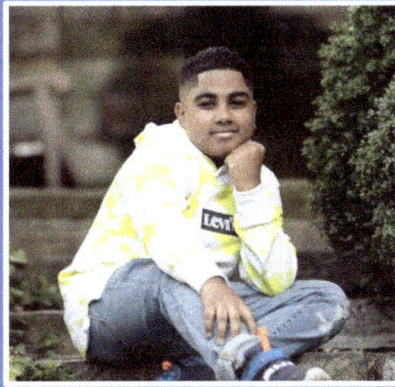

Cristofer is currently a 10 year old multi talented young man with a heart of compassion towards humanity. He is an honor roll student who is gifted in playing musical instruments and great in areas of STEM (Science, Technology, Engineering, Math). He has a special interest in community outreach where he spends a lot of his time helping his mom package food to help struggling families during the pandemic. Cristofer loves playing video games, reading, traveling the world and has an extra love for animals. Someday Cristofer would like to become a veterinarian to help animals around the world and also a computer programmer.

I woke up one morning
and heard Corona was in the air.

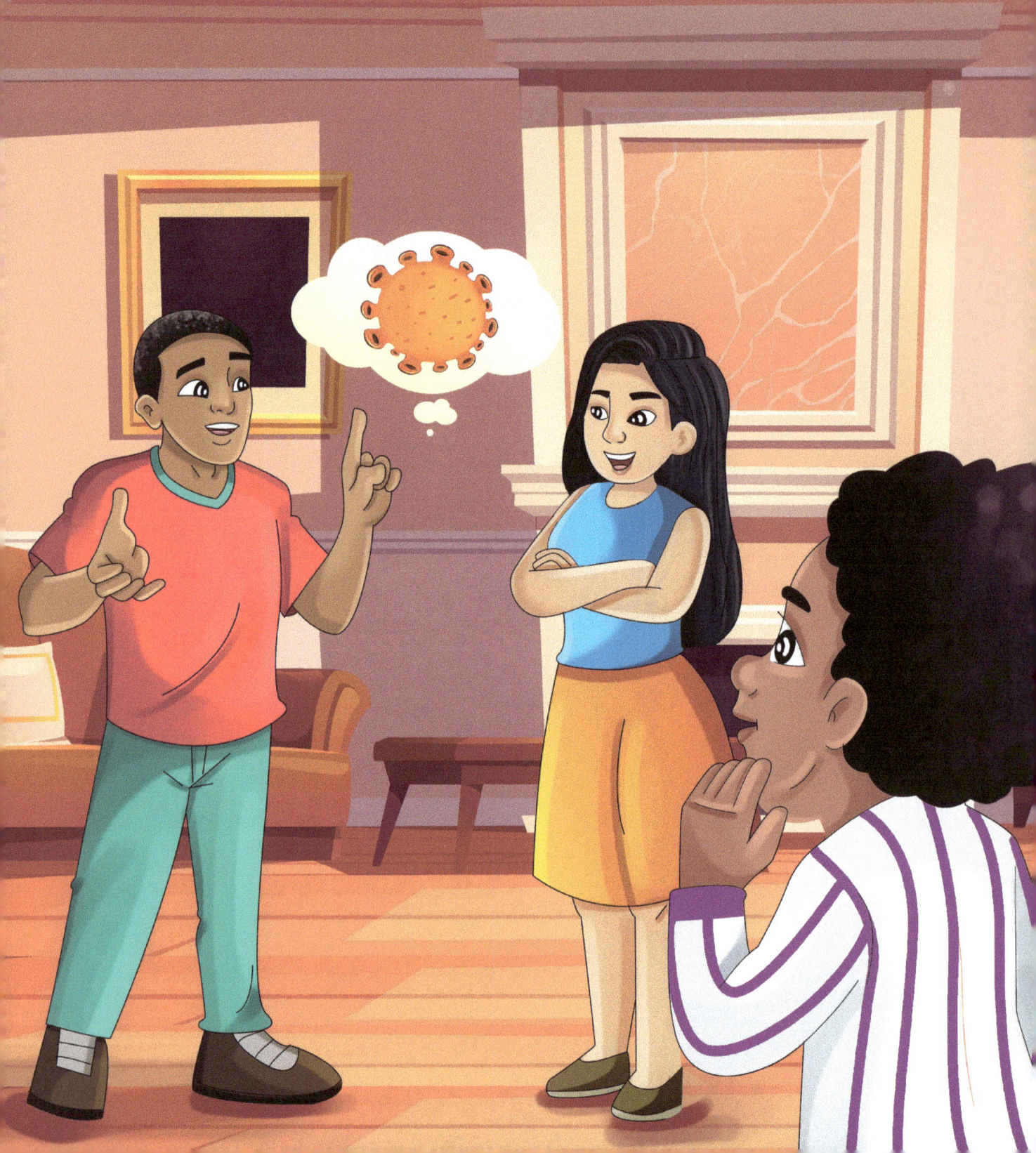

Where did it come from?

At first, no one seemed to care.

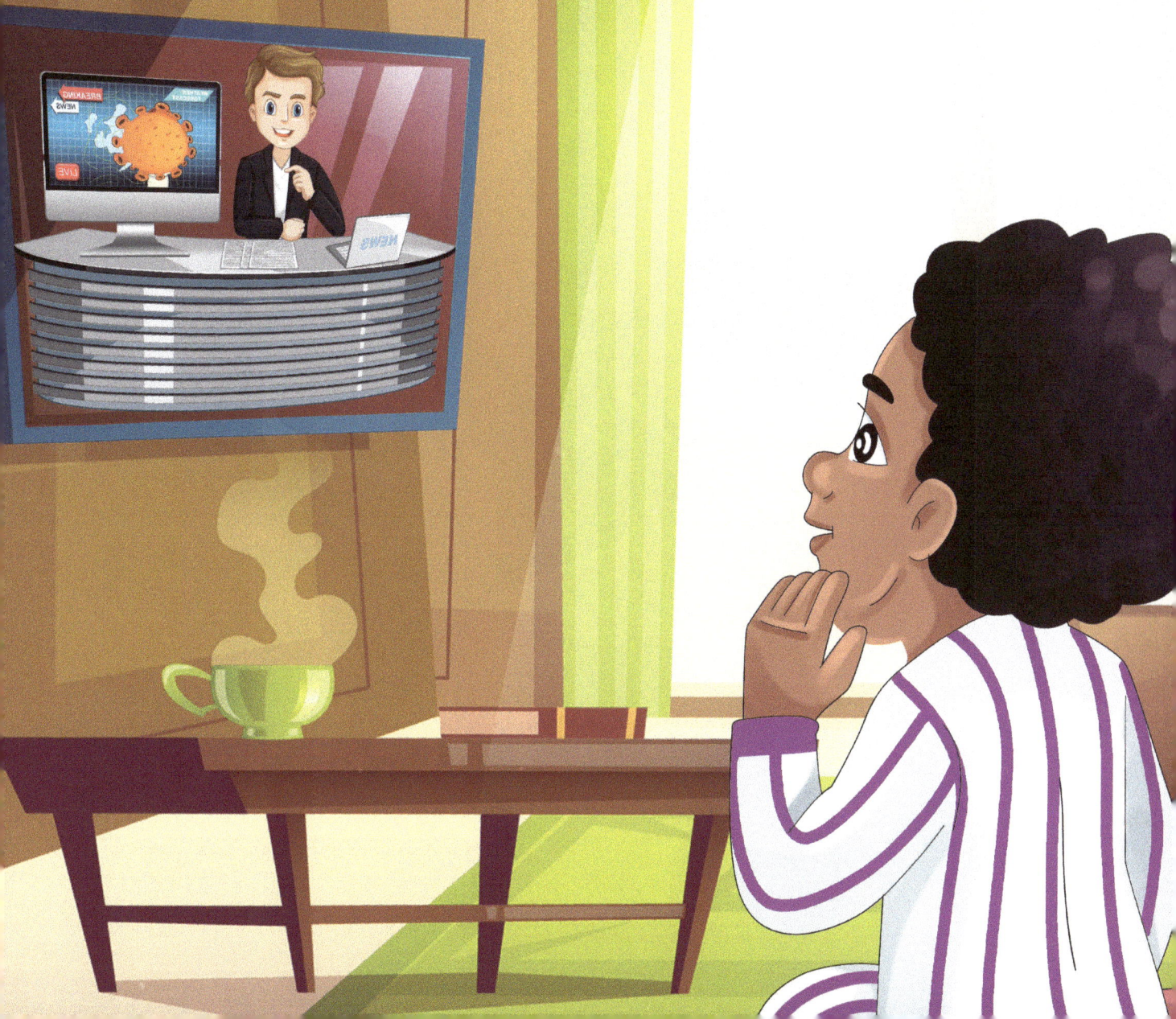

All around the world,
People were seen wearing masks.

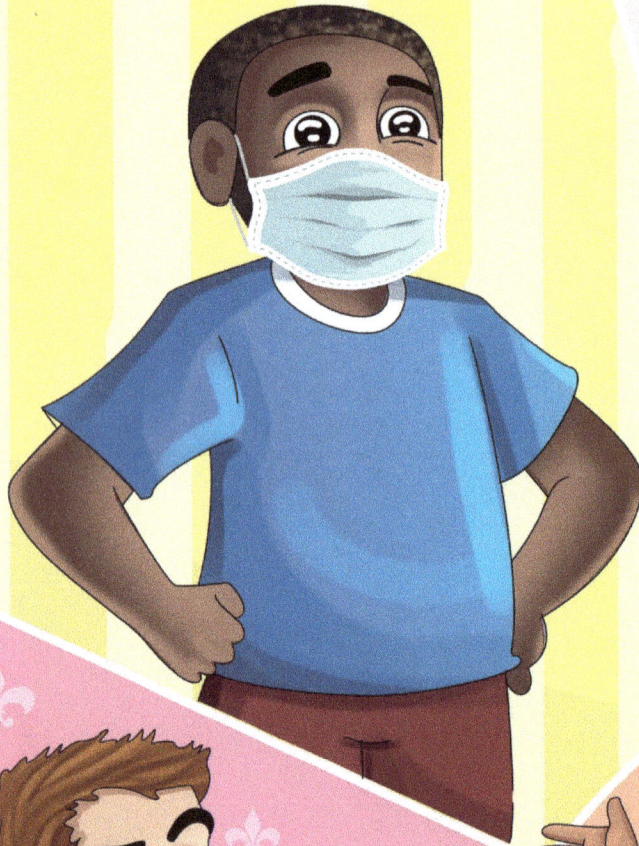

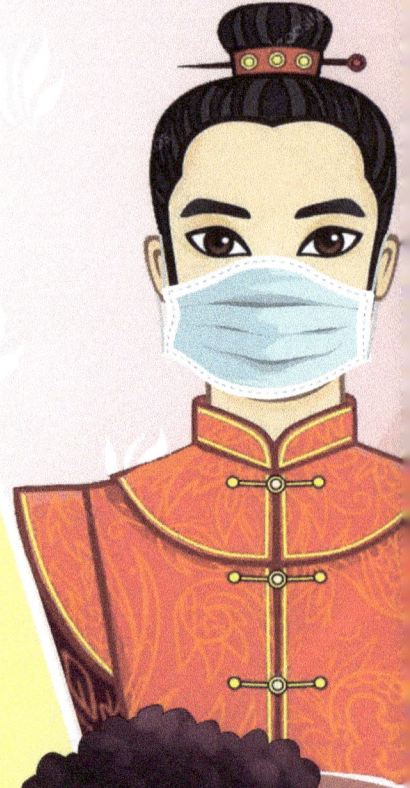

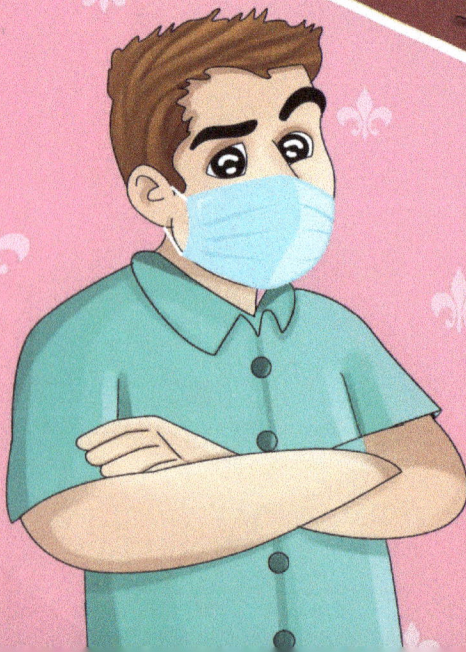

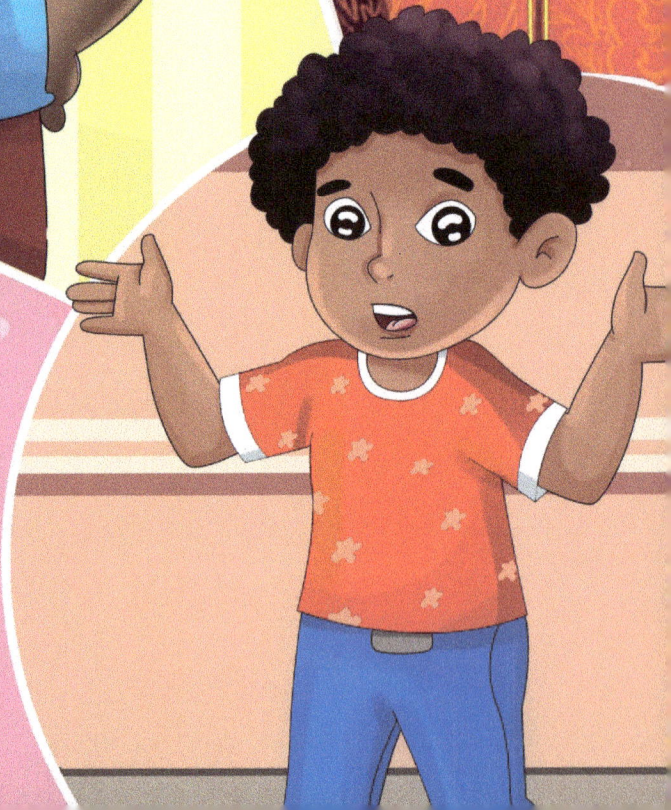

At that point,

I realized I had a list of questions to ask.

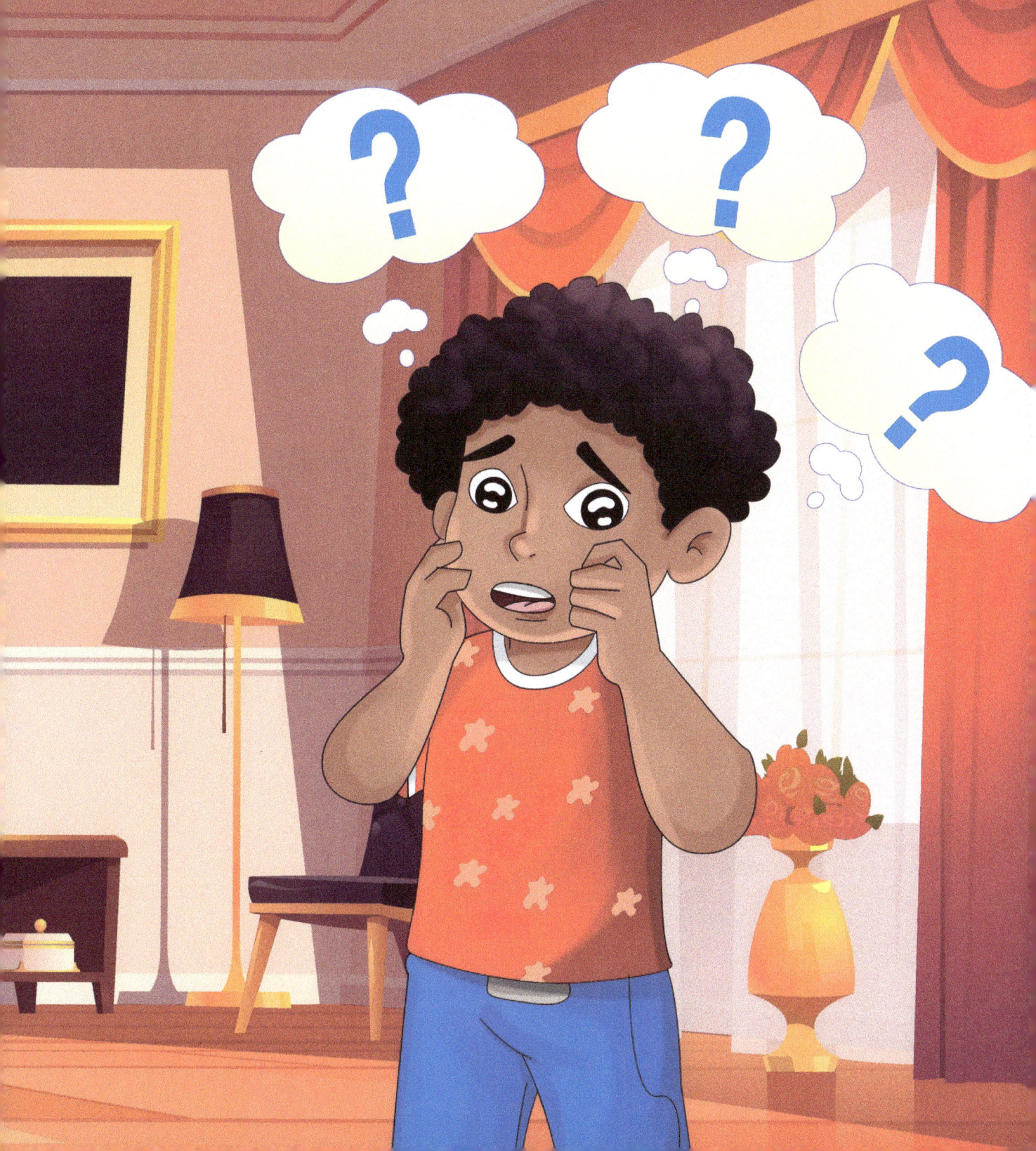

As the days and weeks went by,
Corona looked as if it would never die;

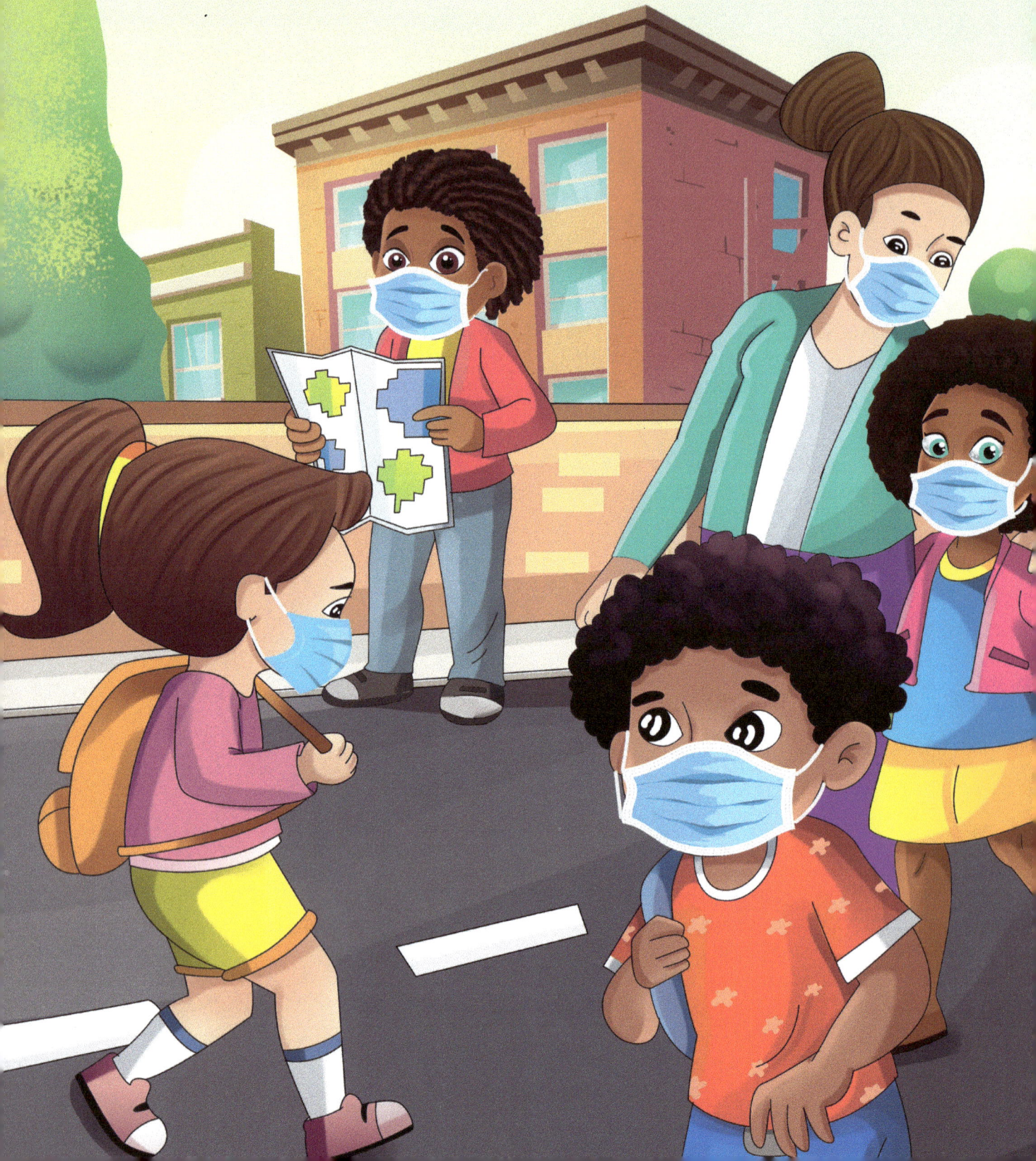

But for a split second, I gazed in the sky,
And said, "Lord, only you know why. "

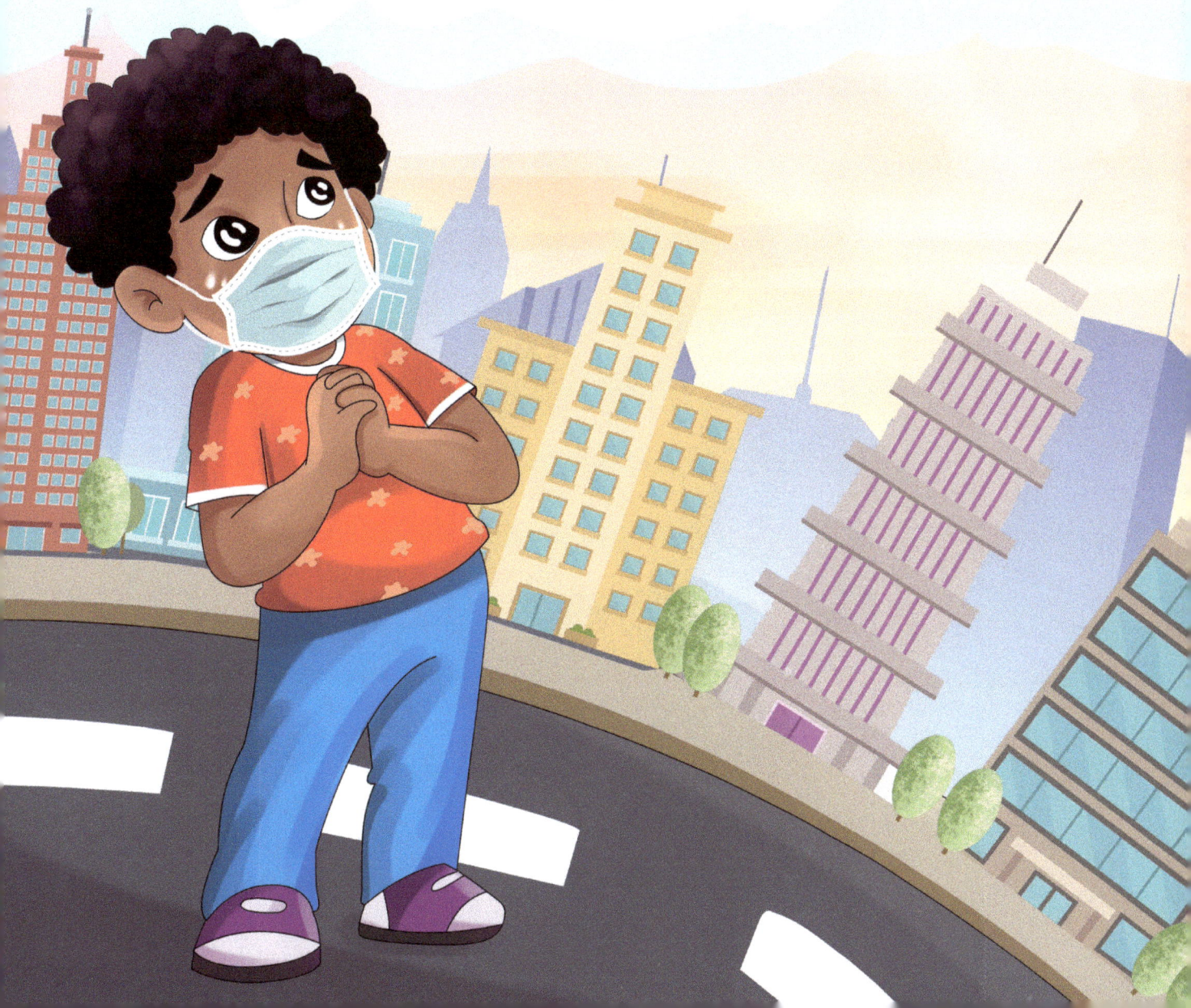

Frontline workers sure do rock!

Those folks were working around the clock.

Busy saving lives here and there,

They must have said, "Corona, please disappear. "

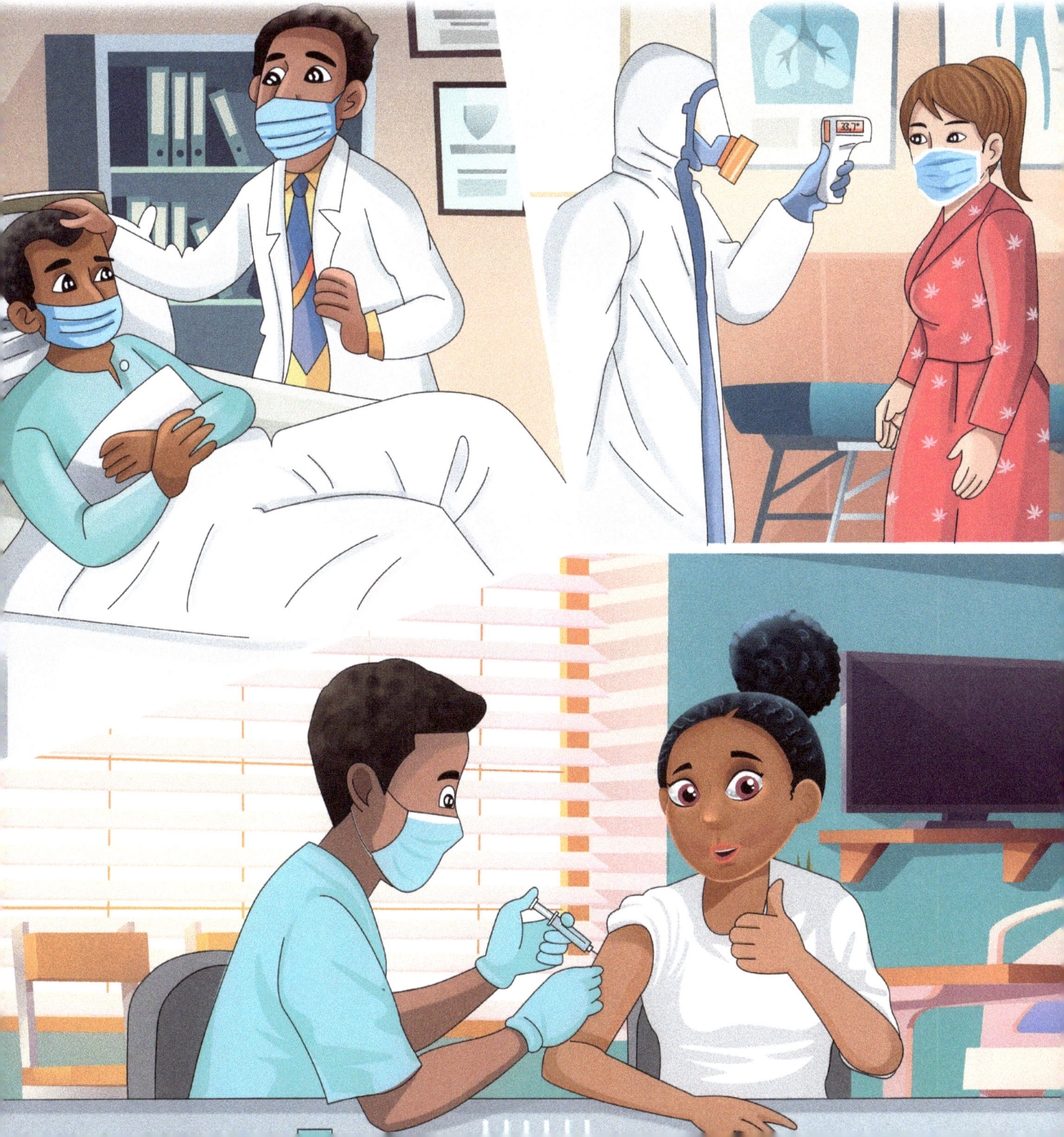

Vacation plans have been cancelled all year.
I noticed Corona was trying hard to bring us fear.

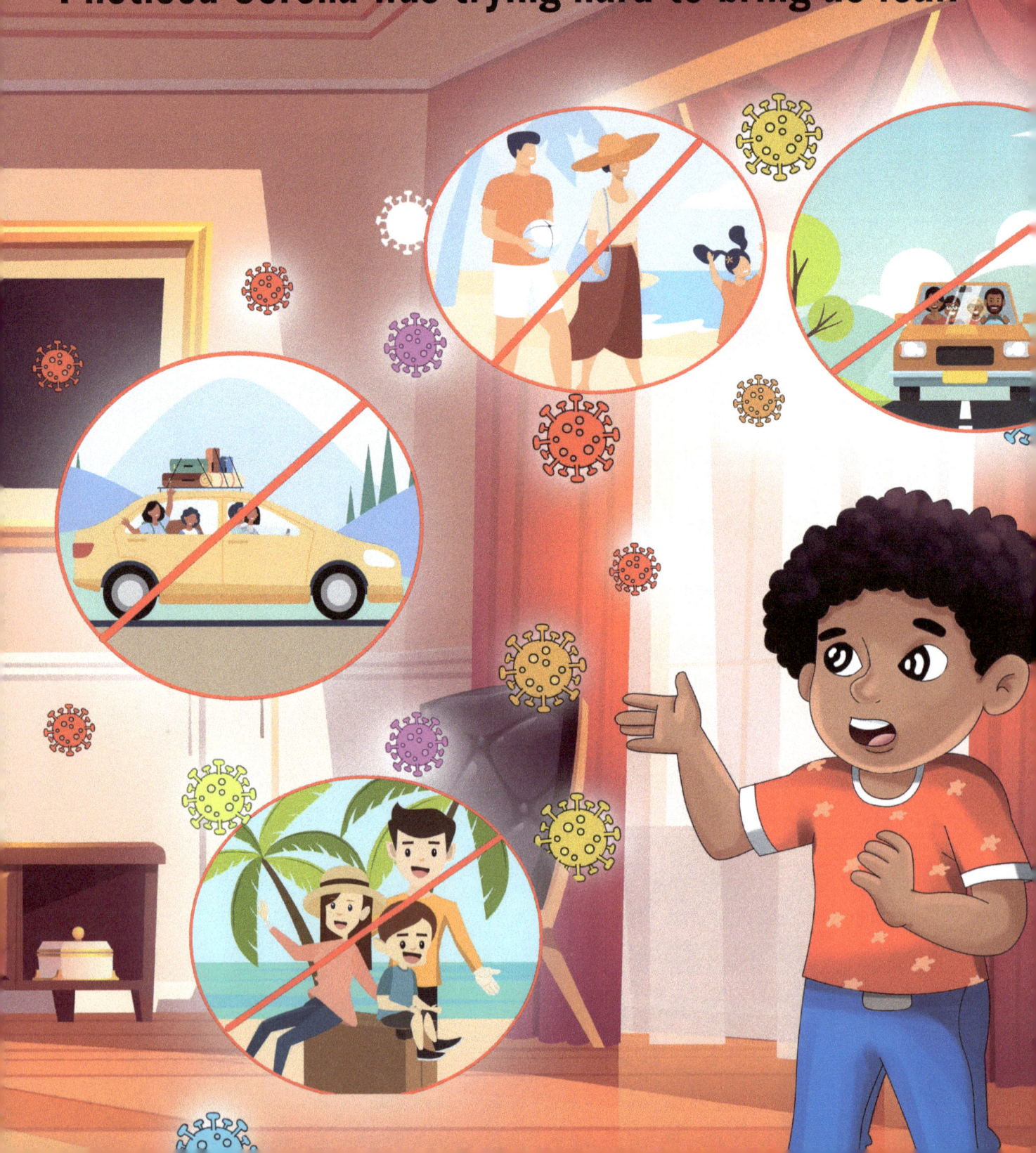

missed my family from Trinidad this summer.

couldn't understand why Corona had to be such a bummer.

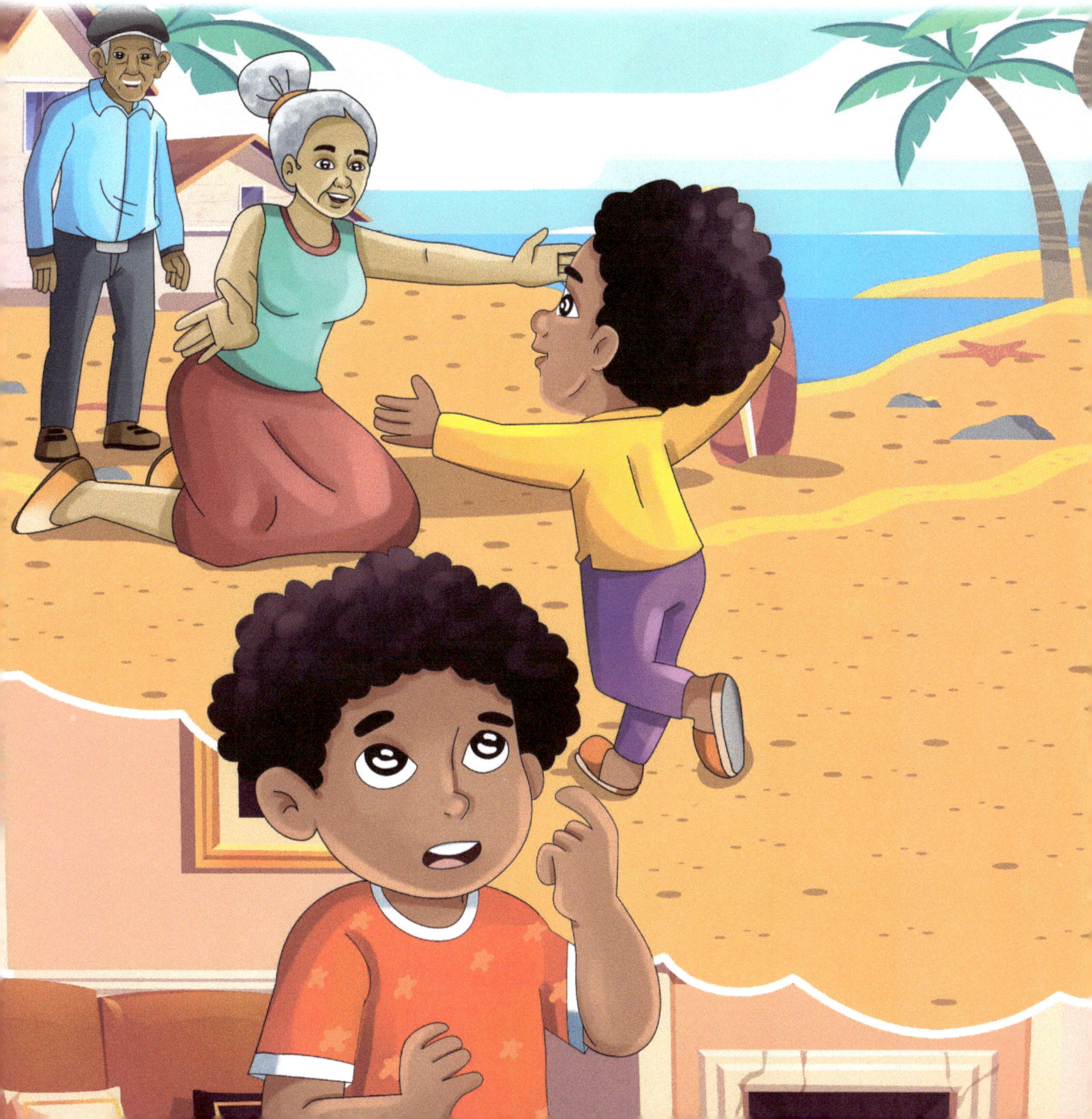

Workers around the world began to sob,
When they found out Corona had affected their jobs.

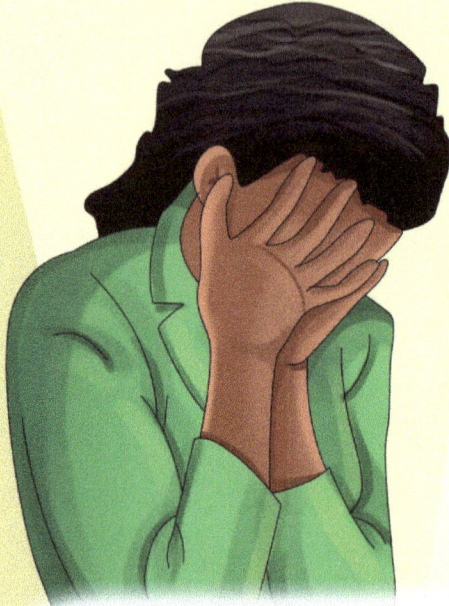
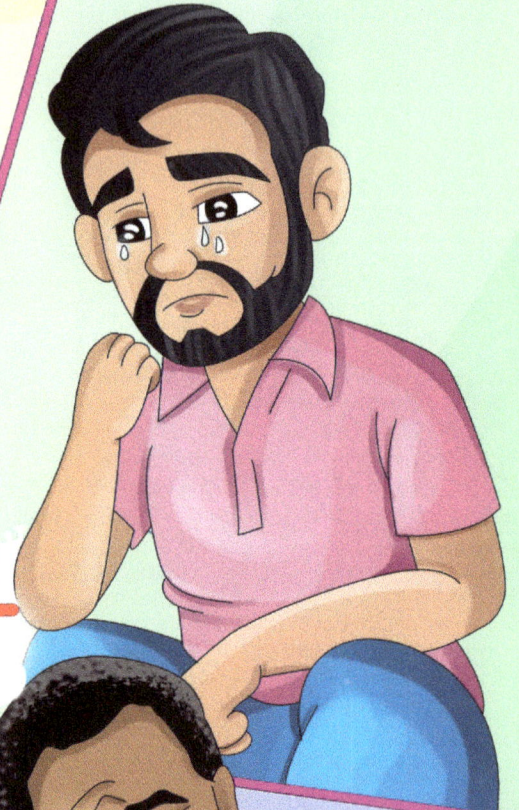
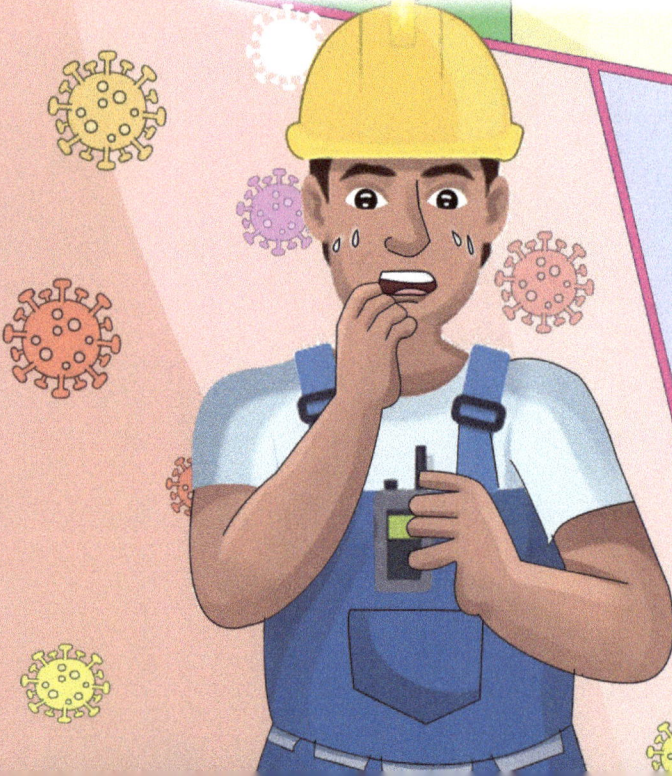
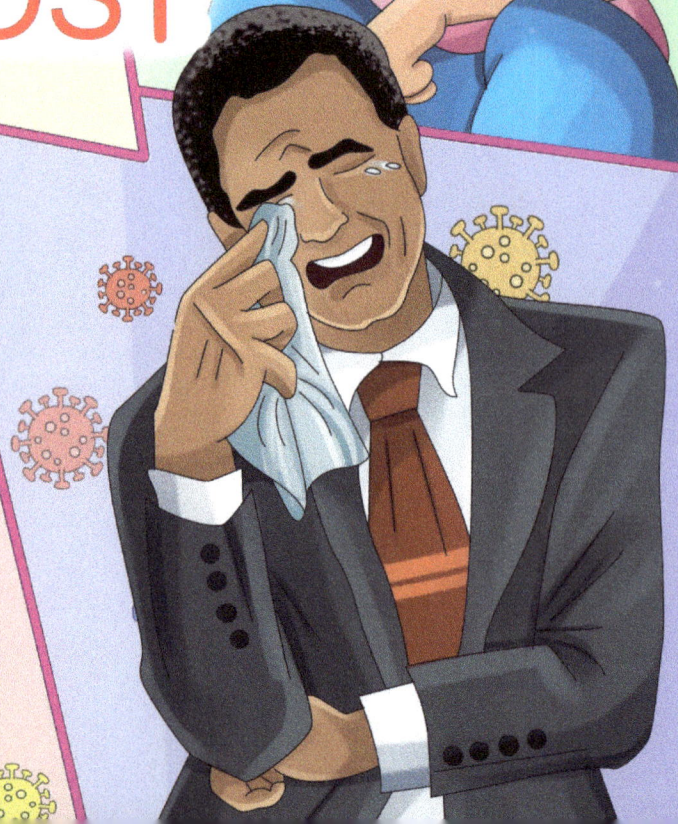

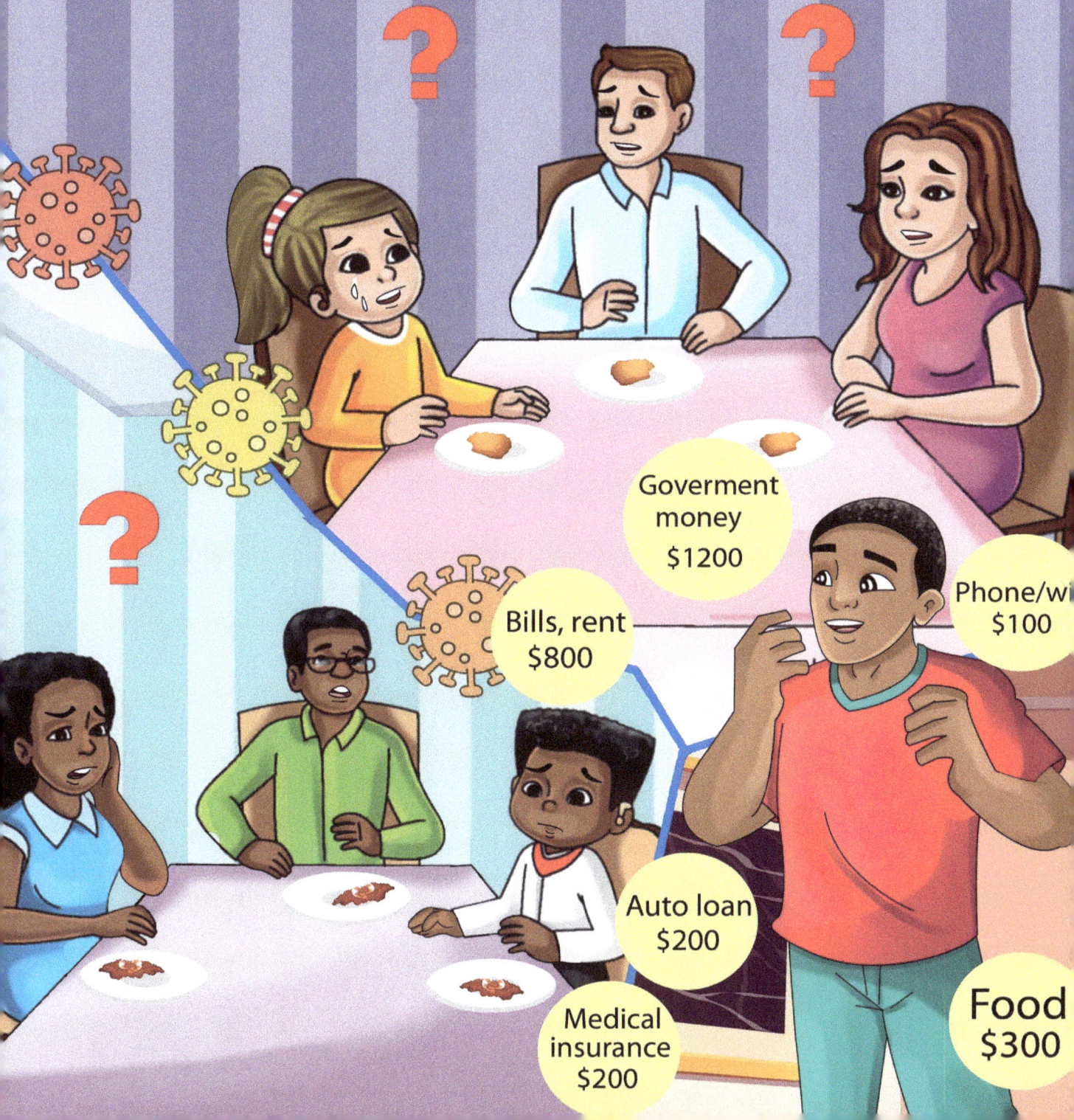

So many families struggled to put food on their table
Even though Congress released a stimulus check,
Many still became unstable.

Schools nationwide suddenly began to close,

As the truth about the deadly virus was exposed.

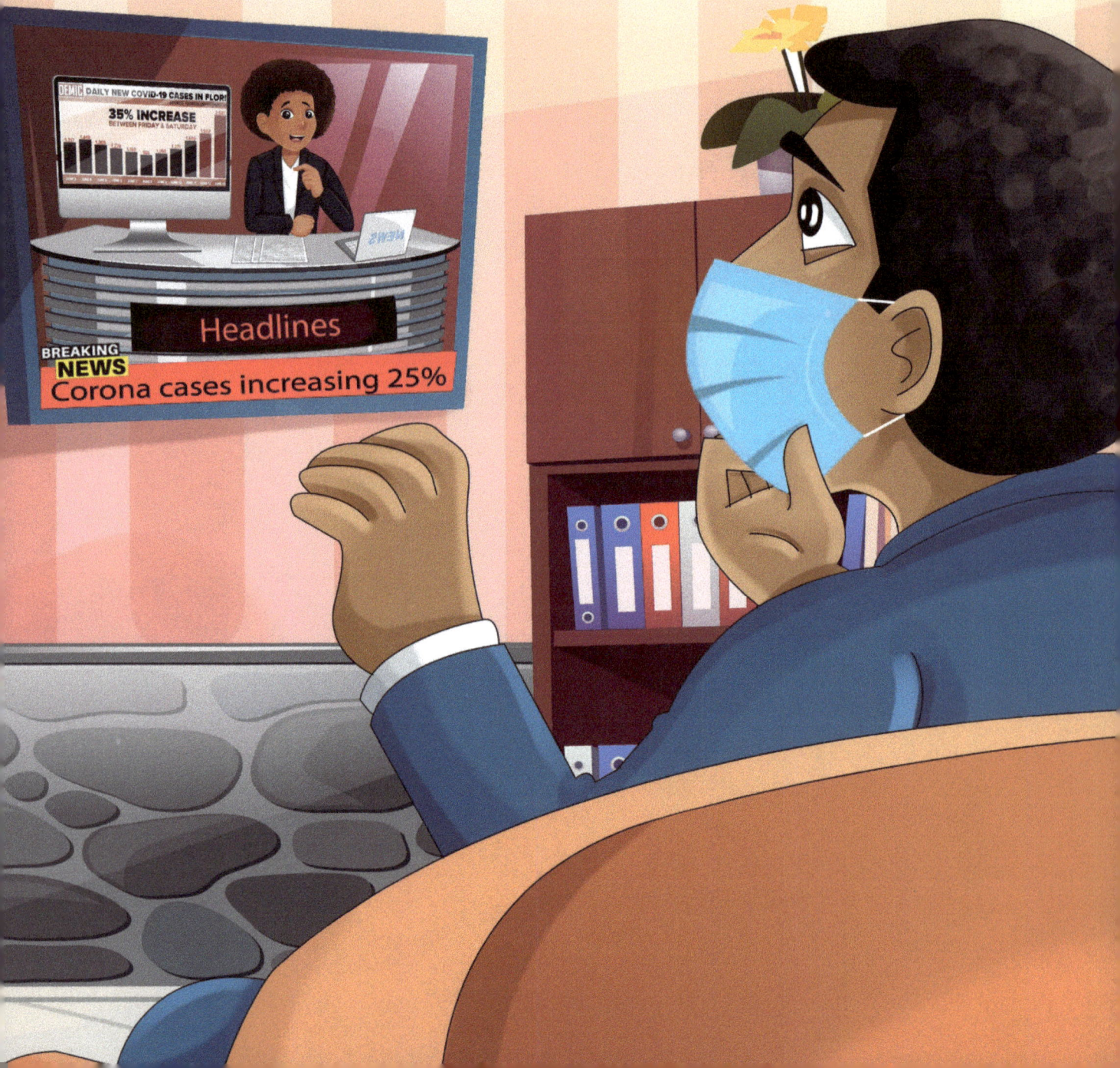

Virtual learning became the new norm,
And parents, teachers, and children took
a while to conform.

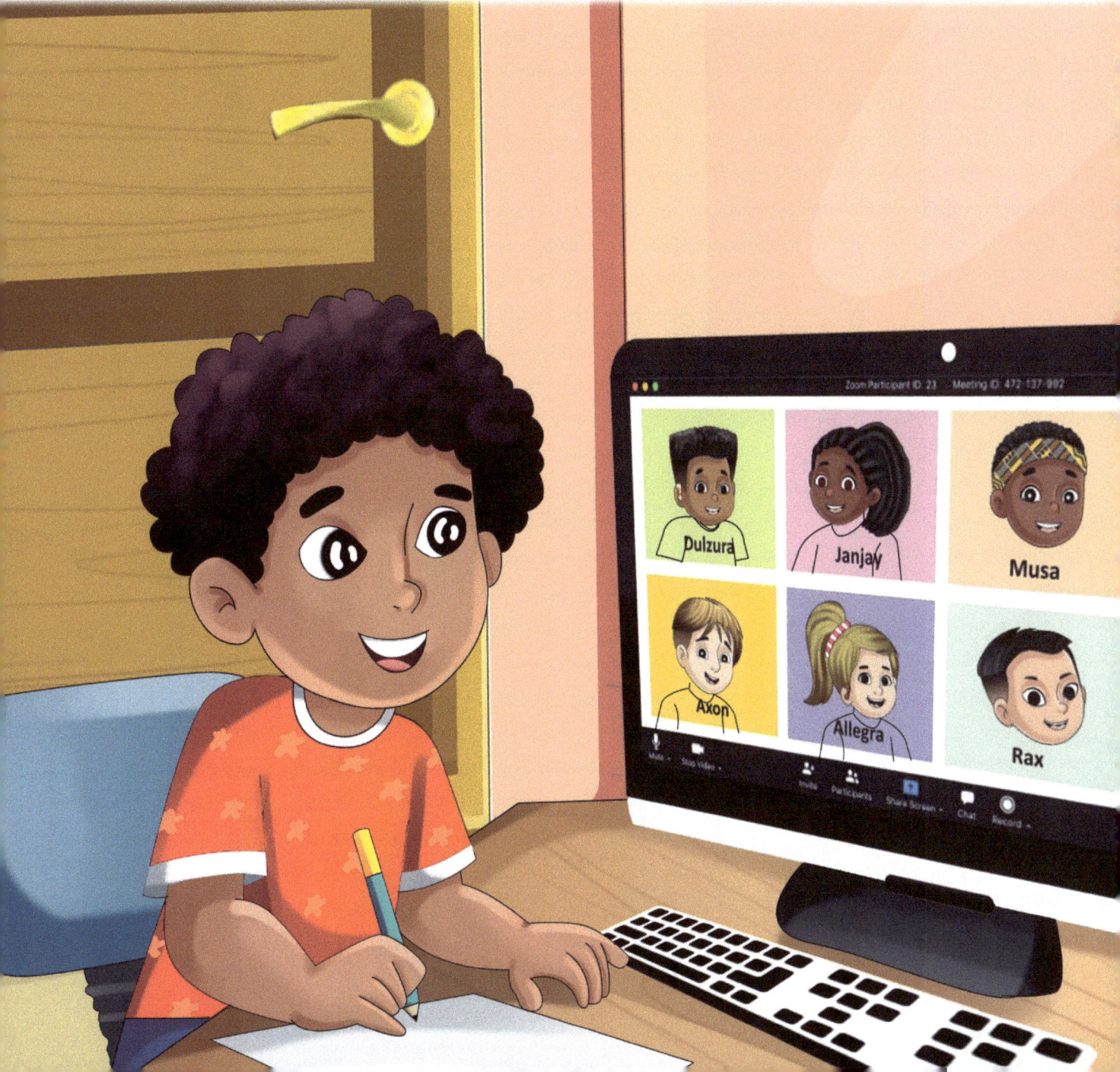

Children had so much fun learning
with friends in schools,
Until Corona showed up, and they all
were sent home to follow new safety rules.

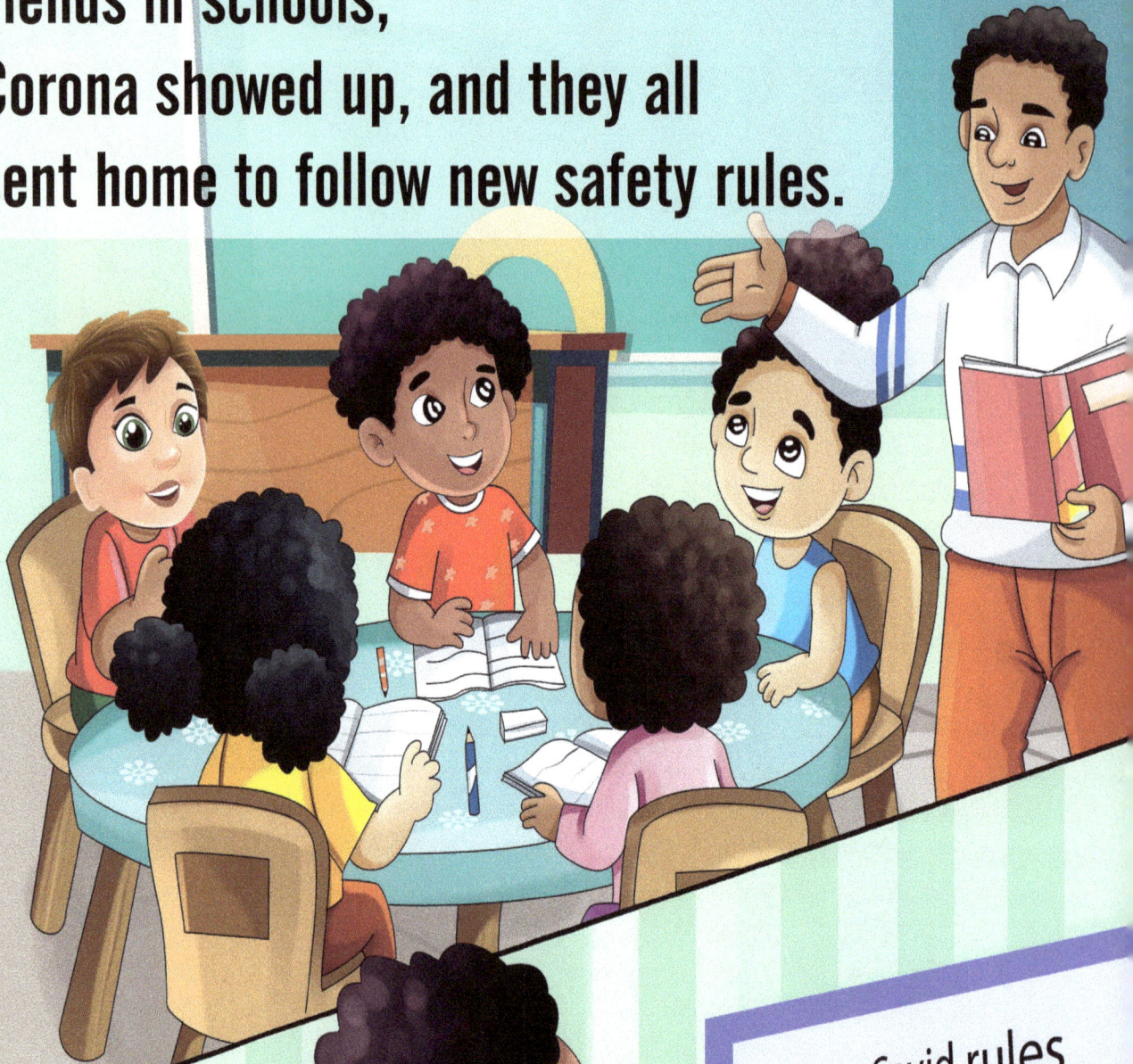

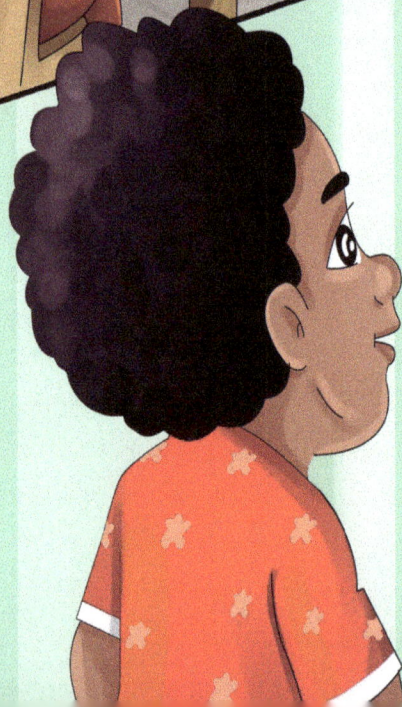

Covid rules

1) Practice social distancin
(6 Feet apart)
2) Wear a mask
3) Wash hands regularly
4) Use hand sanitizer

No more playing tag, hugging, or eating lunch
next to their best friend,
Sadly, all that had to come to an end.

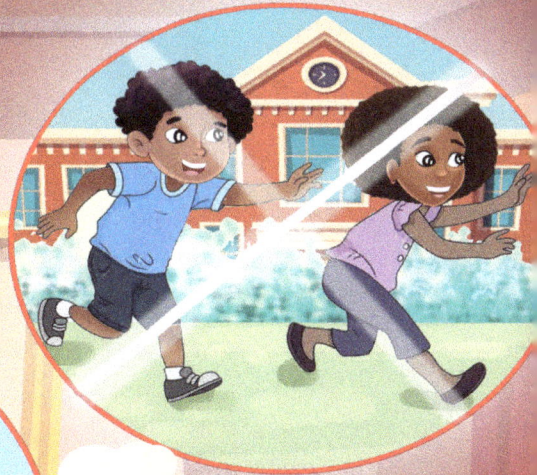
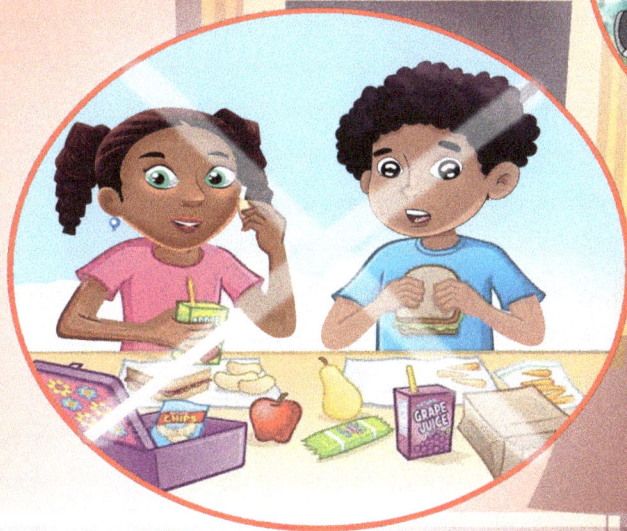
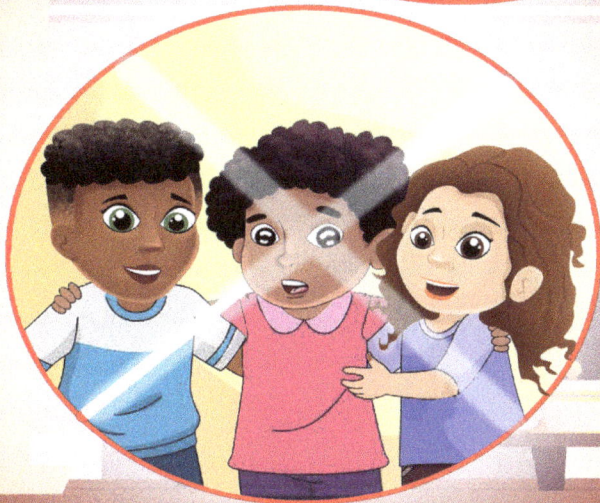
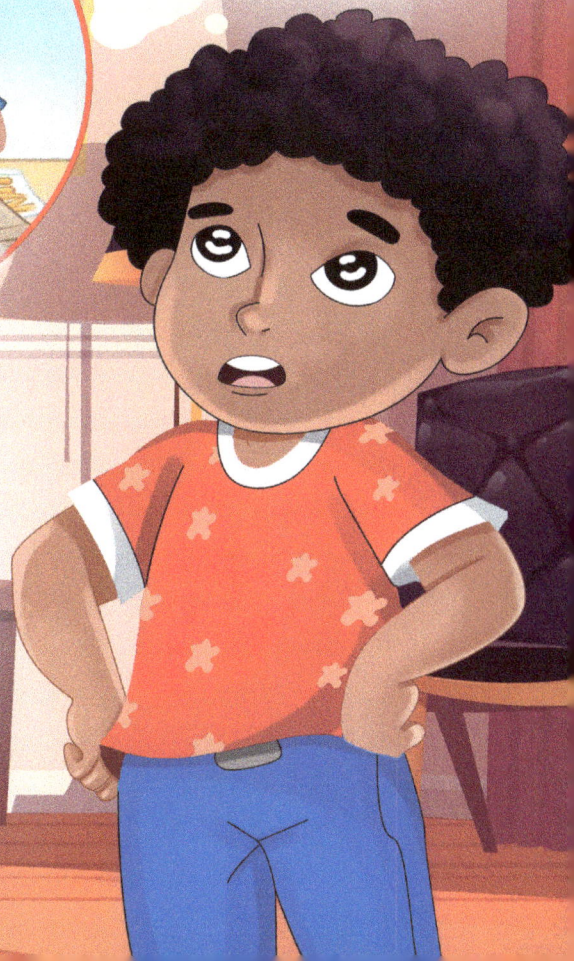

Weddings, birthdays, and funerals all had to be rushed. Plans for Thanksgiving feasts and other holidays were suddenly crushed.

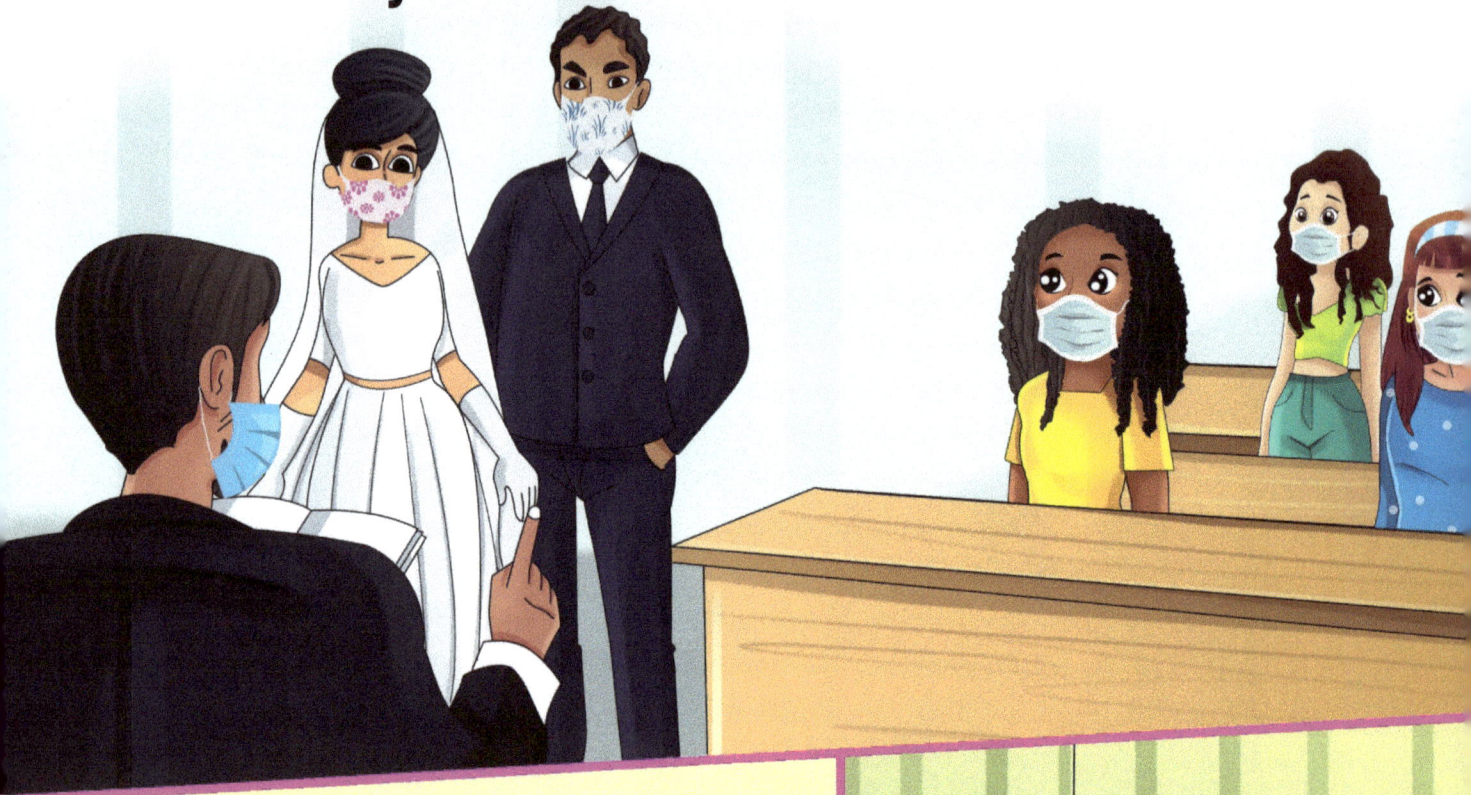

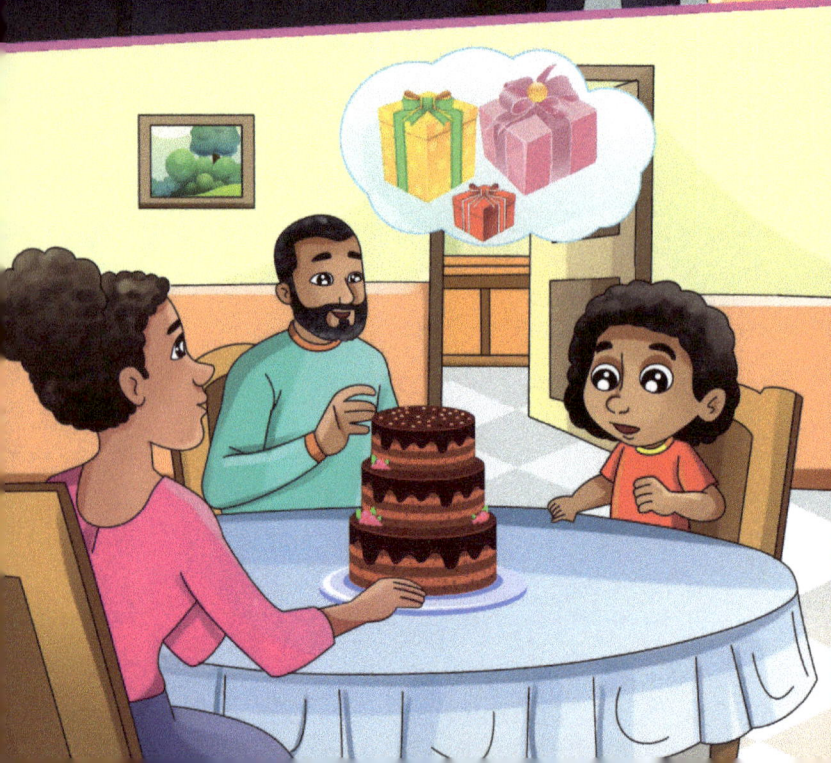

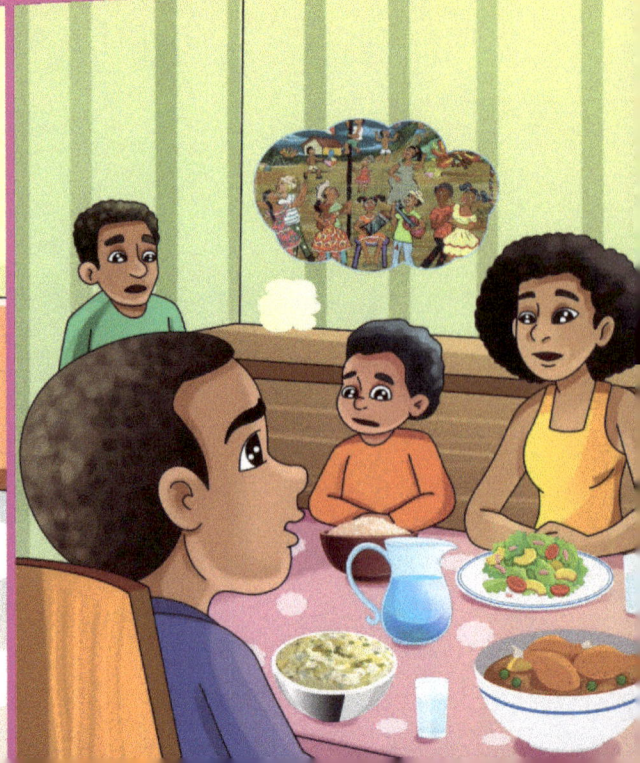

Corona caused so many restrictions worldwide,
In most places, only ten or fewer could gather inside.

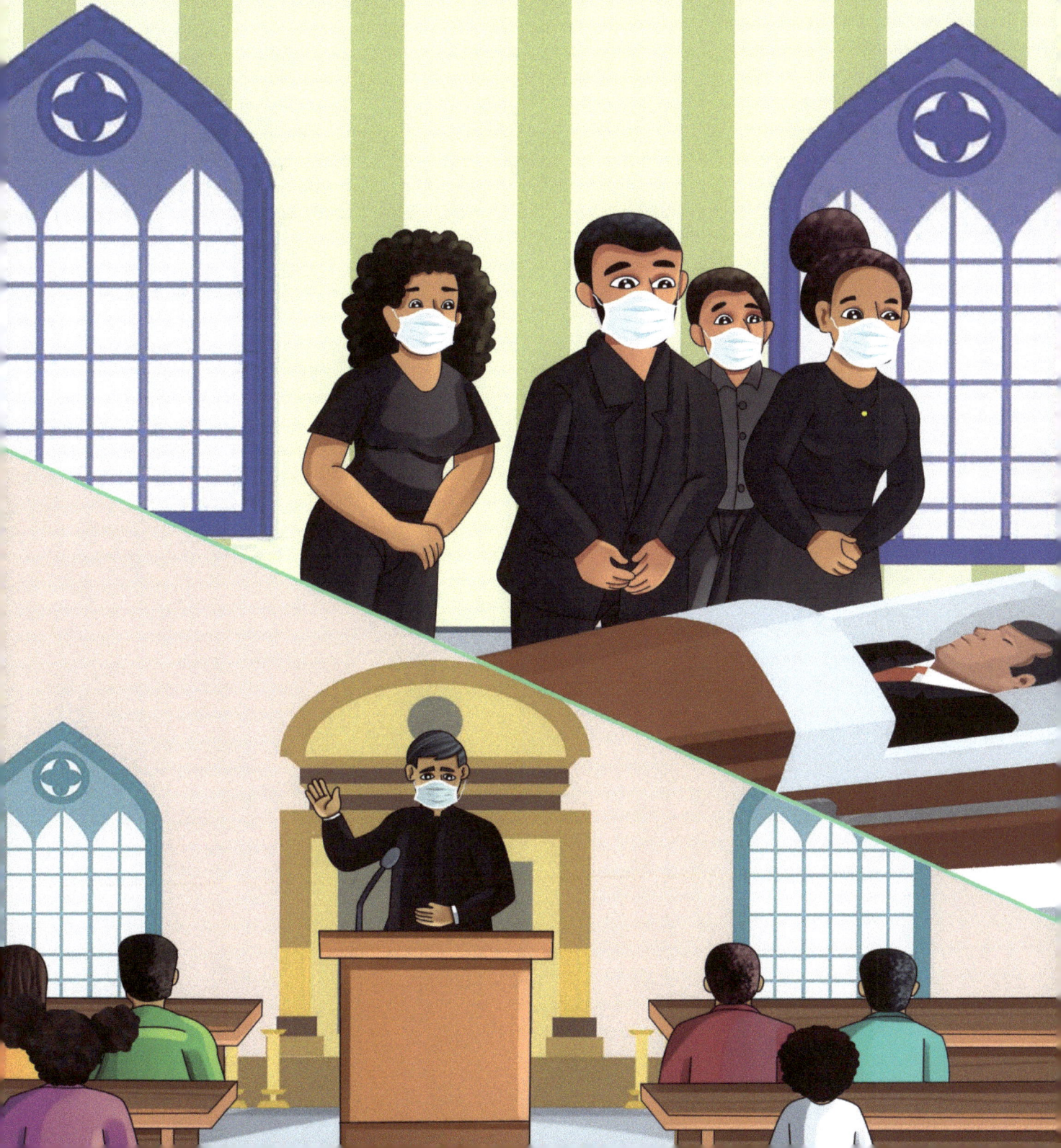

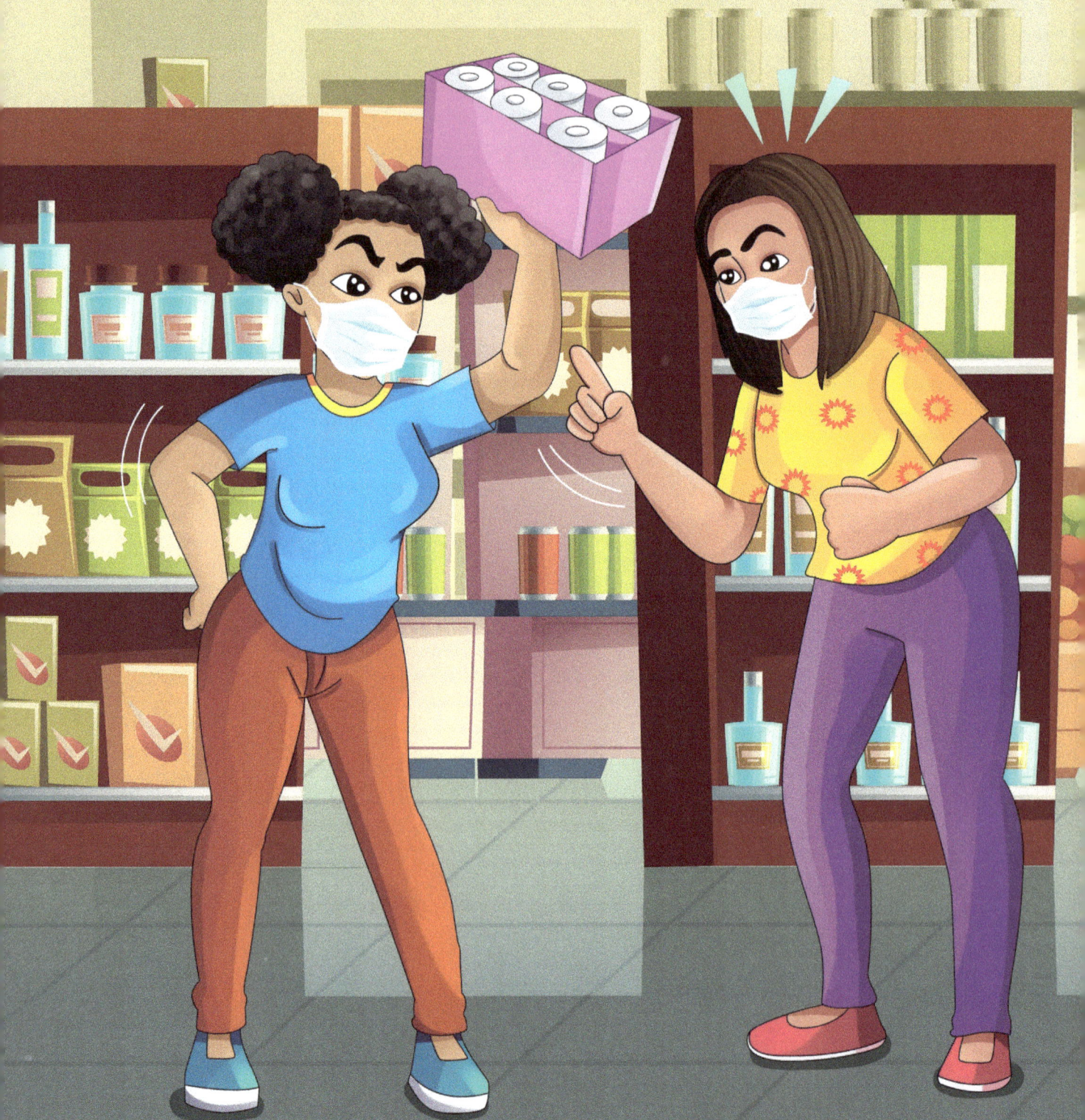

Not to mention how angry people felt searching for Lysol and toilet paper tissue.

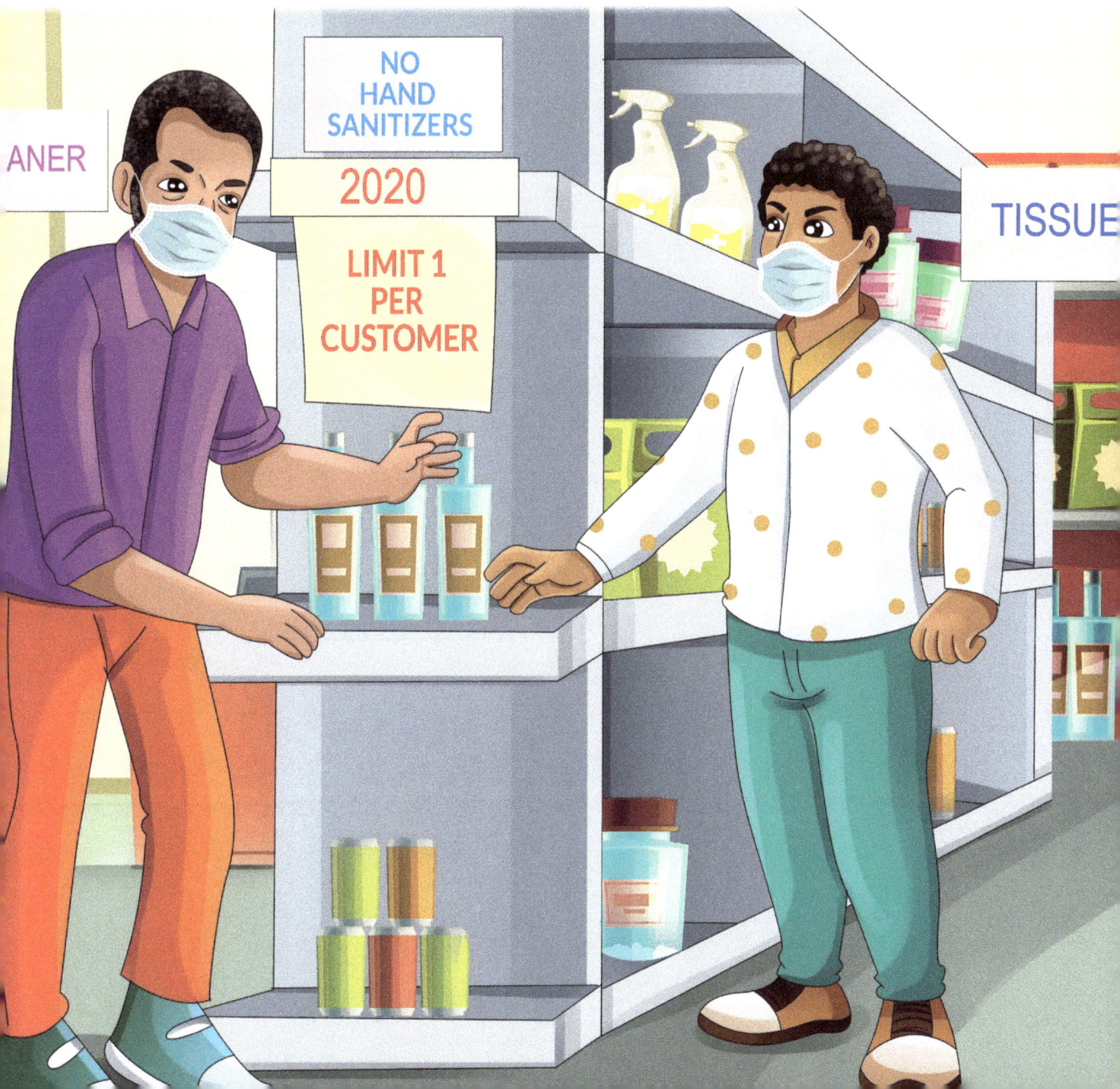

But despite how chaotic the world seemed,
Corona brought out hidden talents
of which many had dreamed.

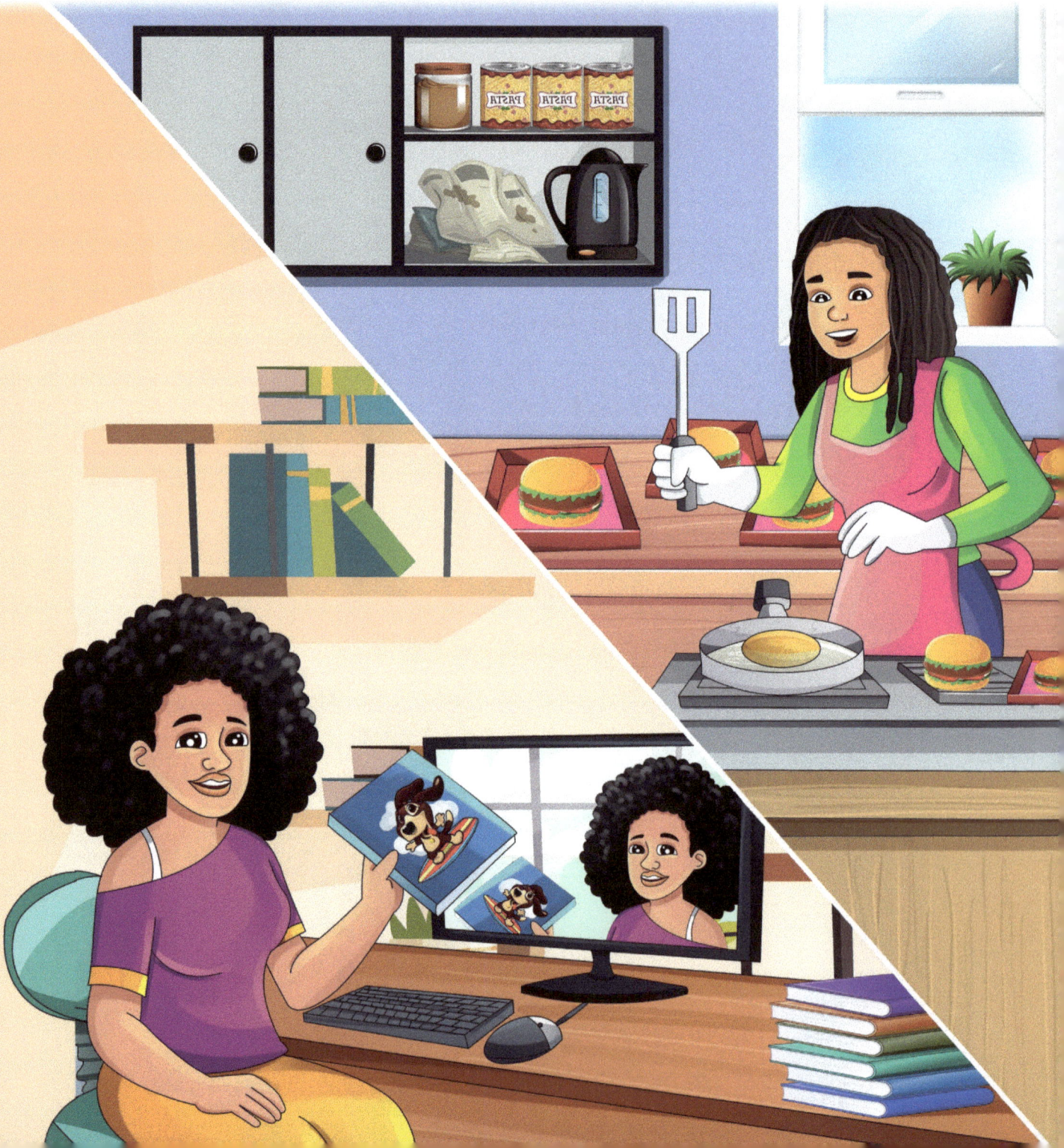

From sewing masks and selling food,
Corona had people doing business online
in a hopeful mood.

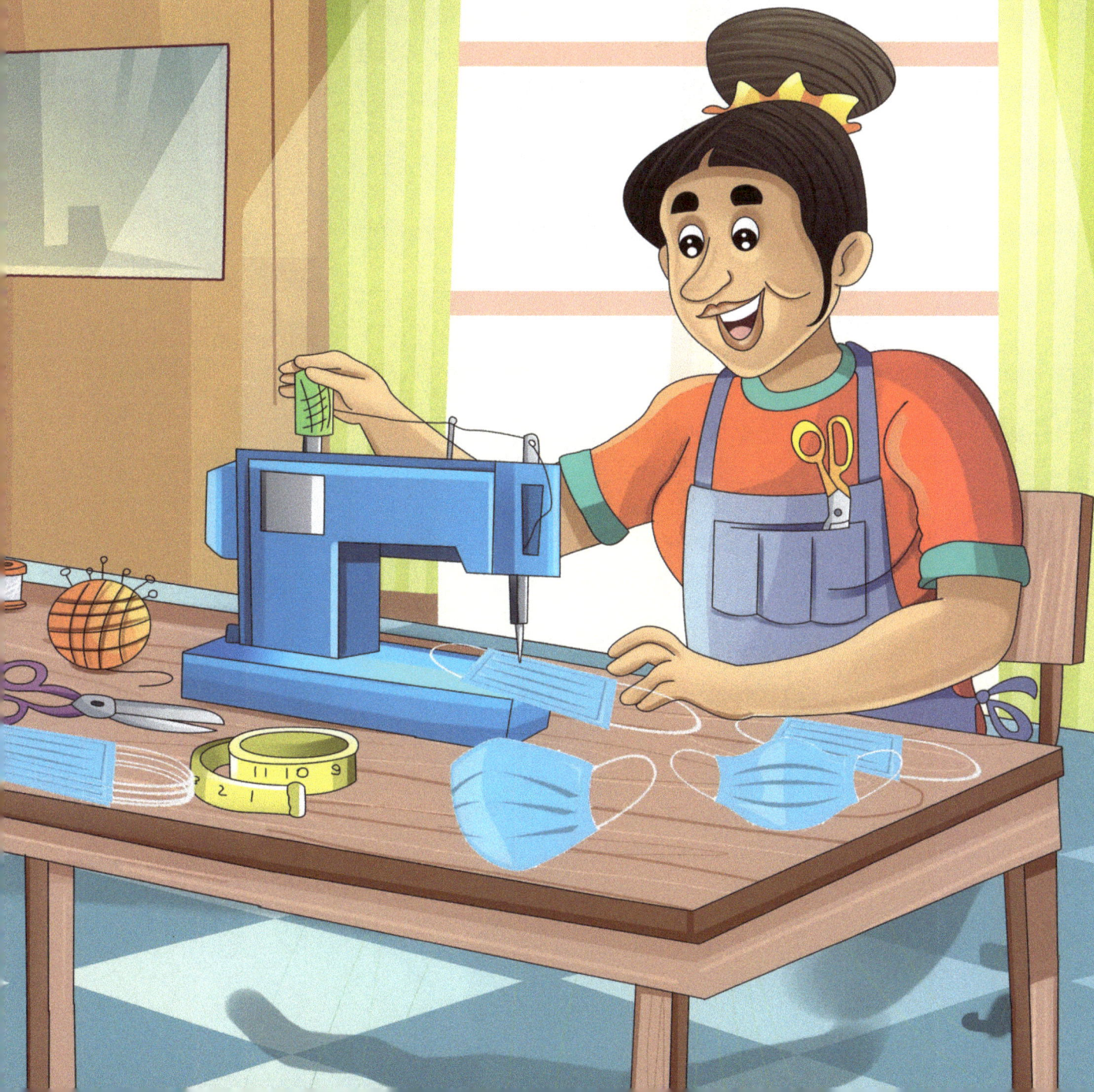

Families were spreading love together once more,
Since Corona kept many parents from rushing out the door.

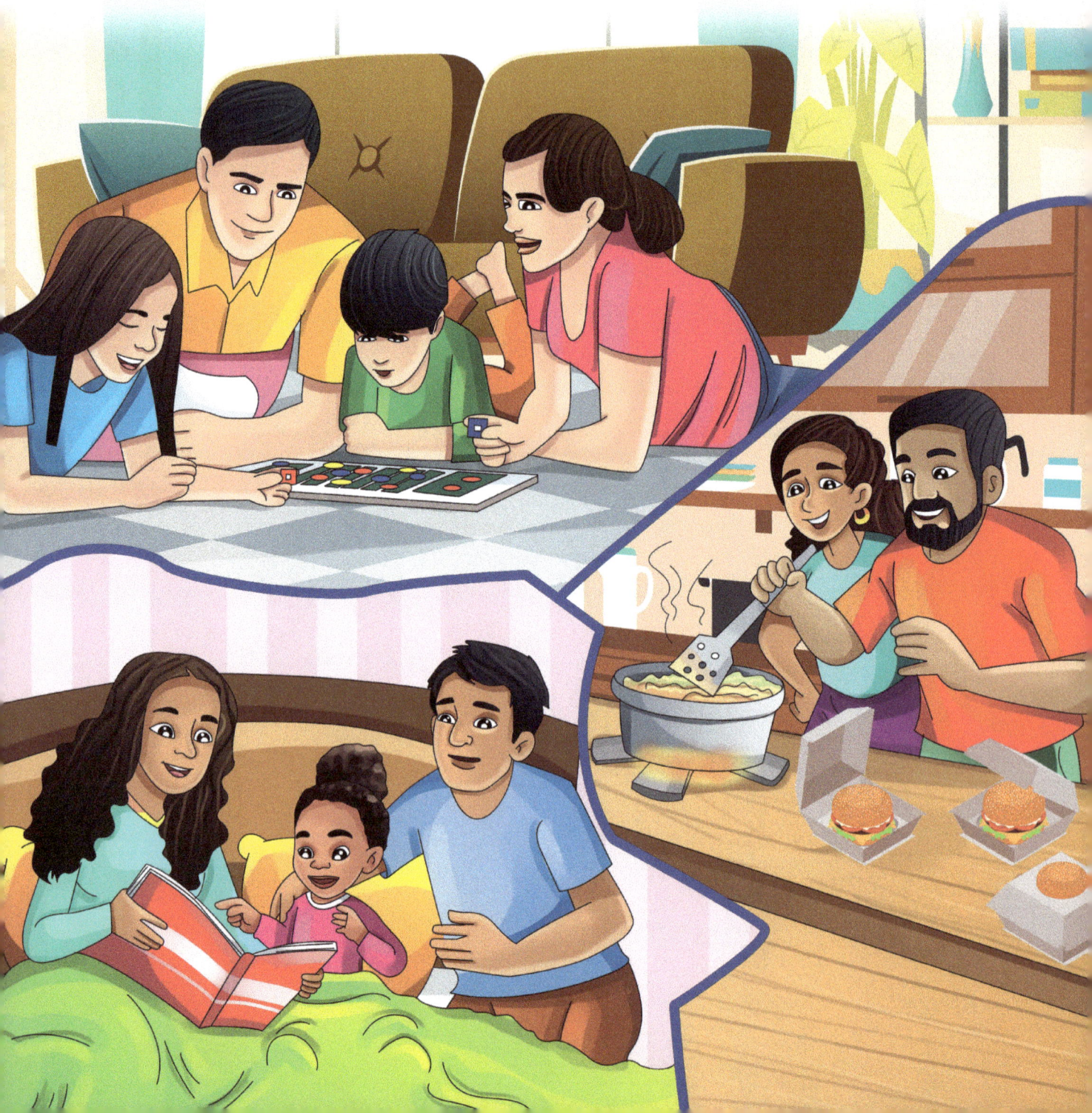

Many were focused on lending support,
When they realized how life can be short.

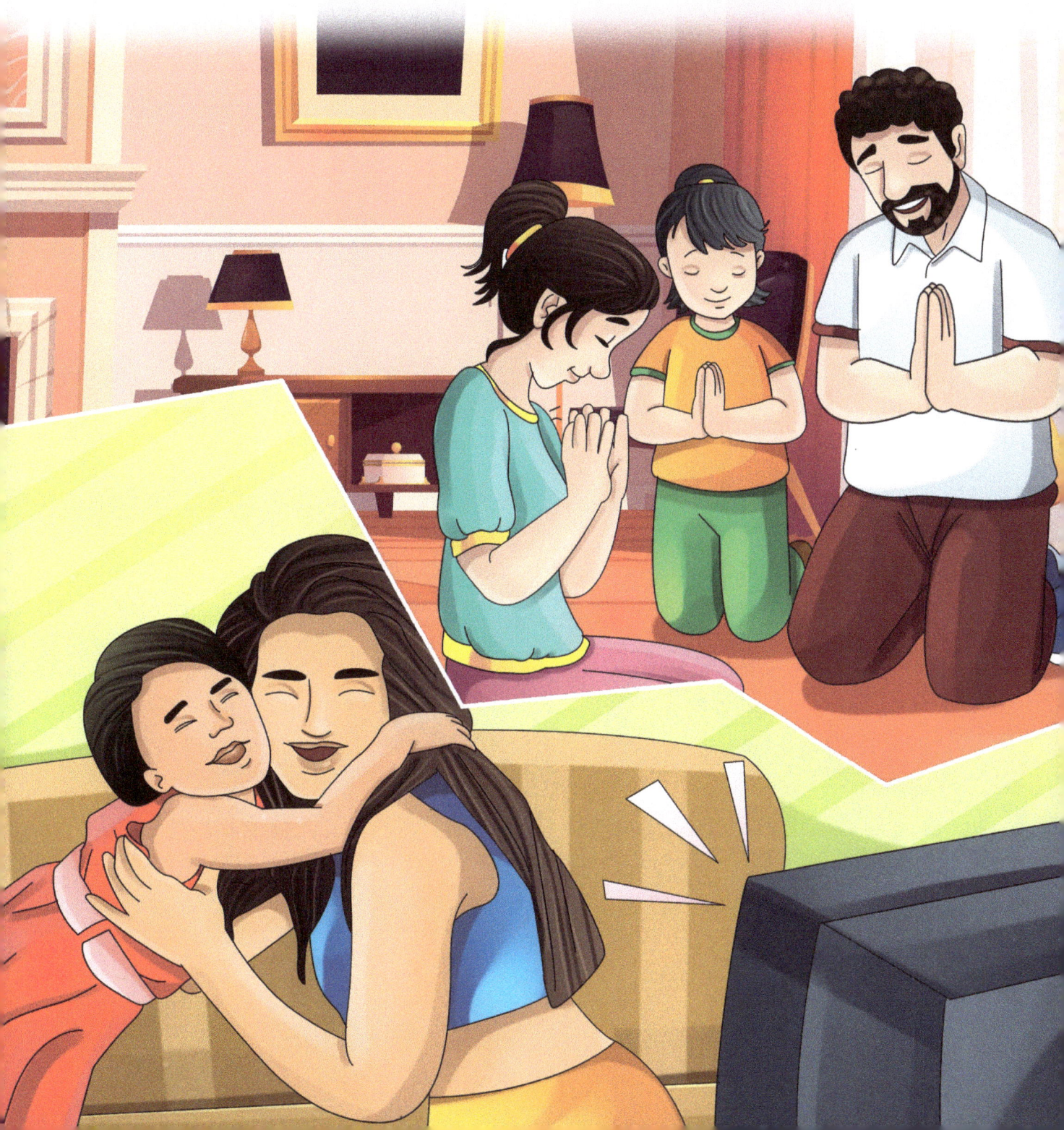

Corona had more people reaching out for prayer,
Hoping the end of the world was not near.

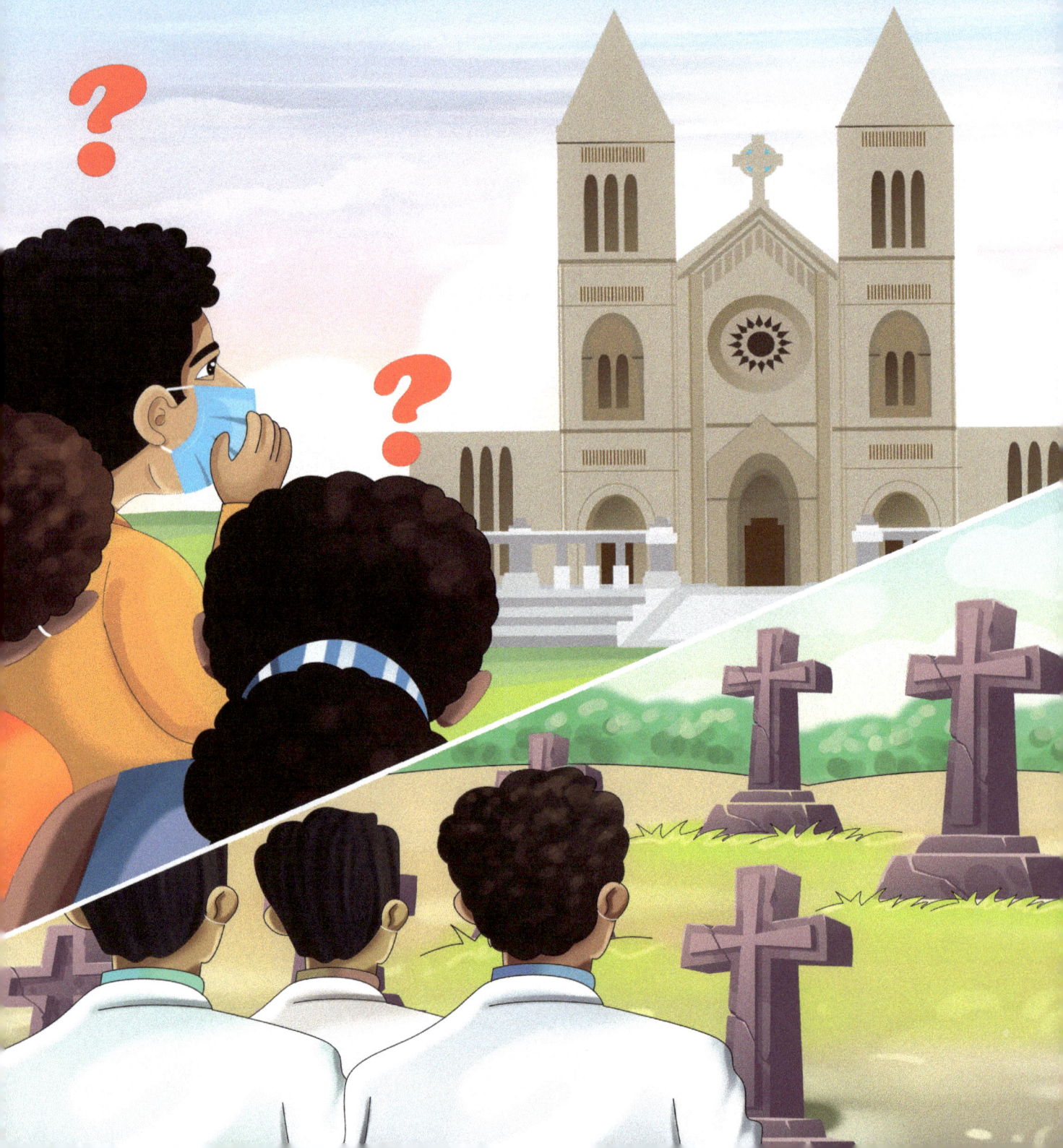

Thankfully, the church was prepared,
And demonstrated how much they cared.
Sharing food here and there,
With healing miracles happening everywhere.

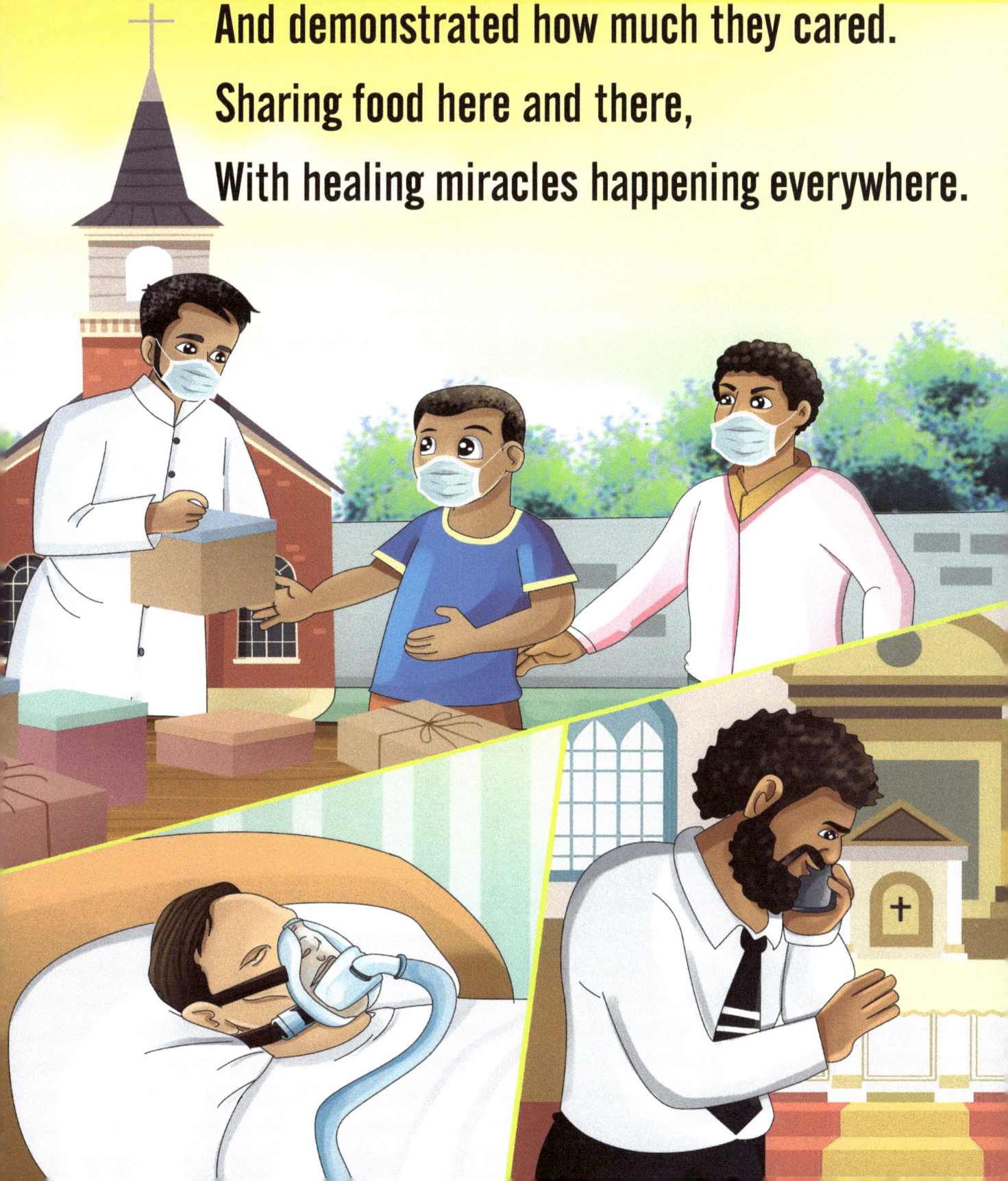

Then came a heated election,
With many demonstrating hate
from just a projection.

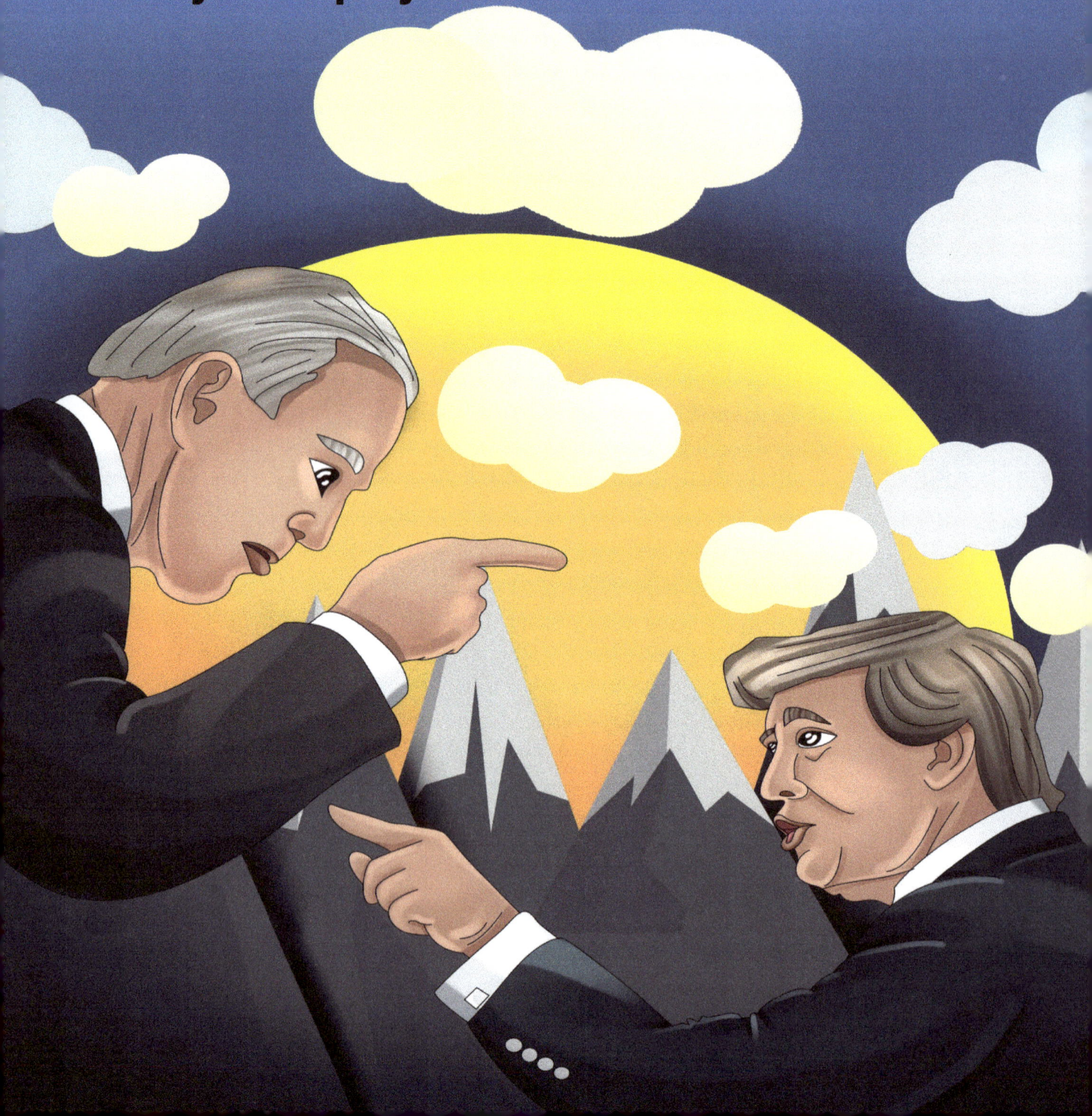

Angry armed supporters stormed Capitol Hill,
Venting their anger to impose their own will.

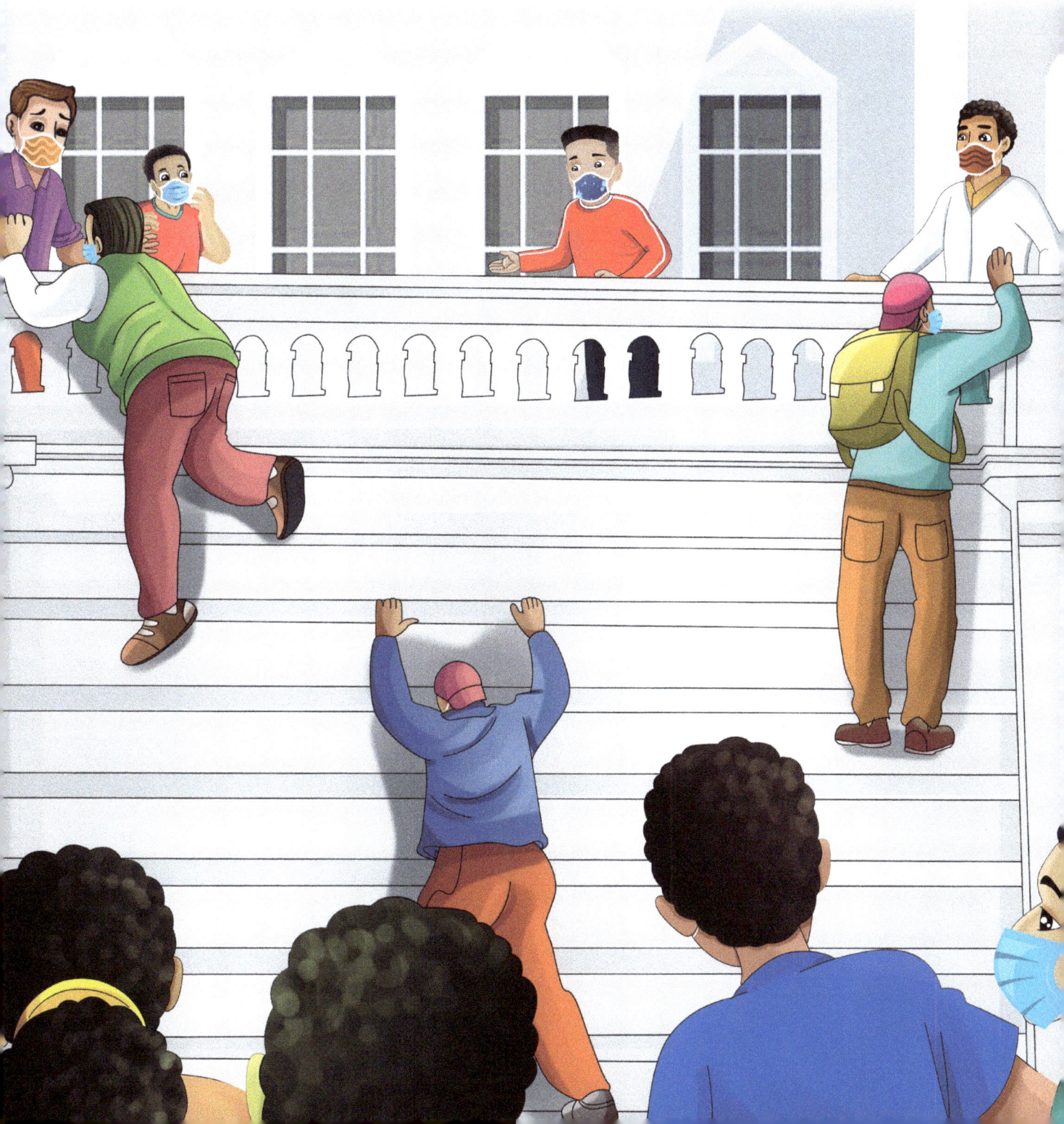

Even as the end of the year was near,
Corona still seemed to be in the air.

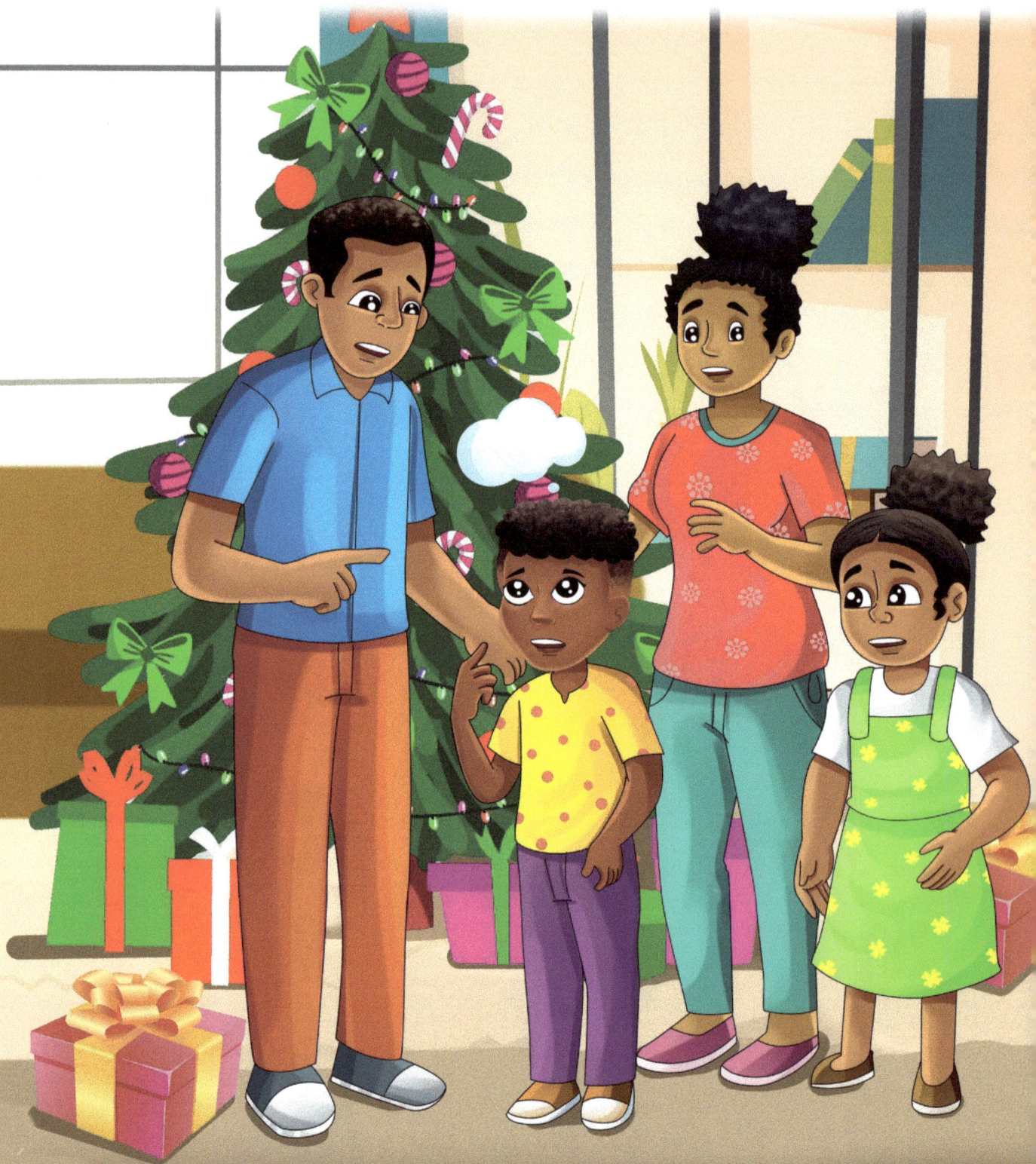

Rumors of new vaccines were finally out,
Yet, many were still in doubt.

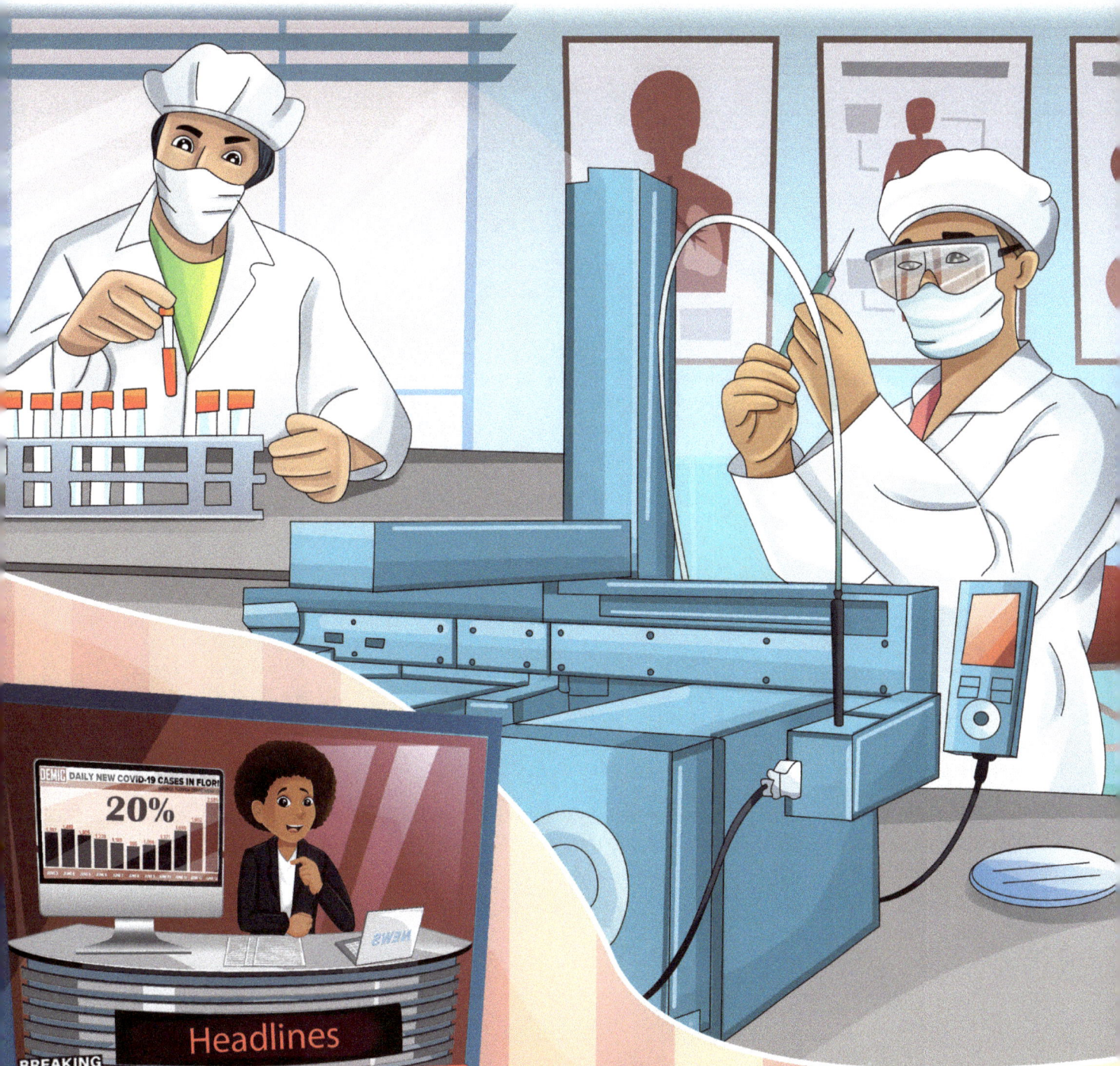

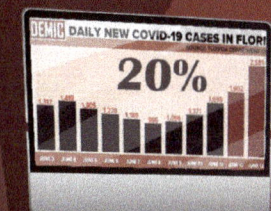

"How long again before Corona ends?"
Was the question volleyed back
and forth amongst many friends.

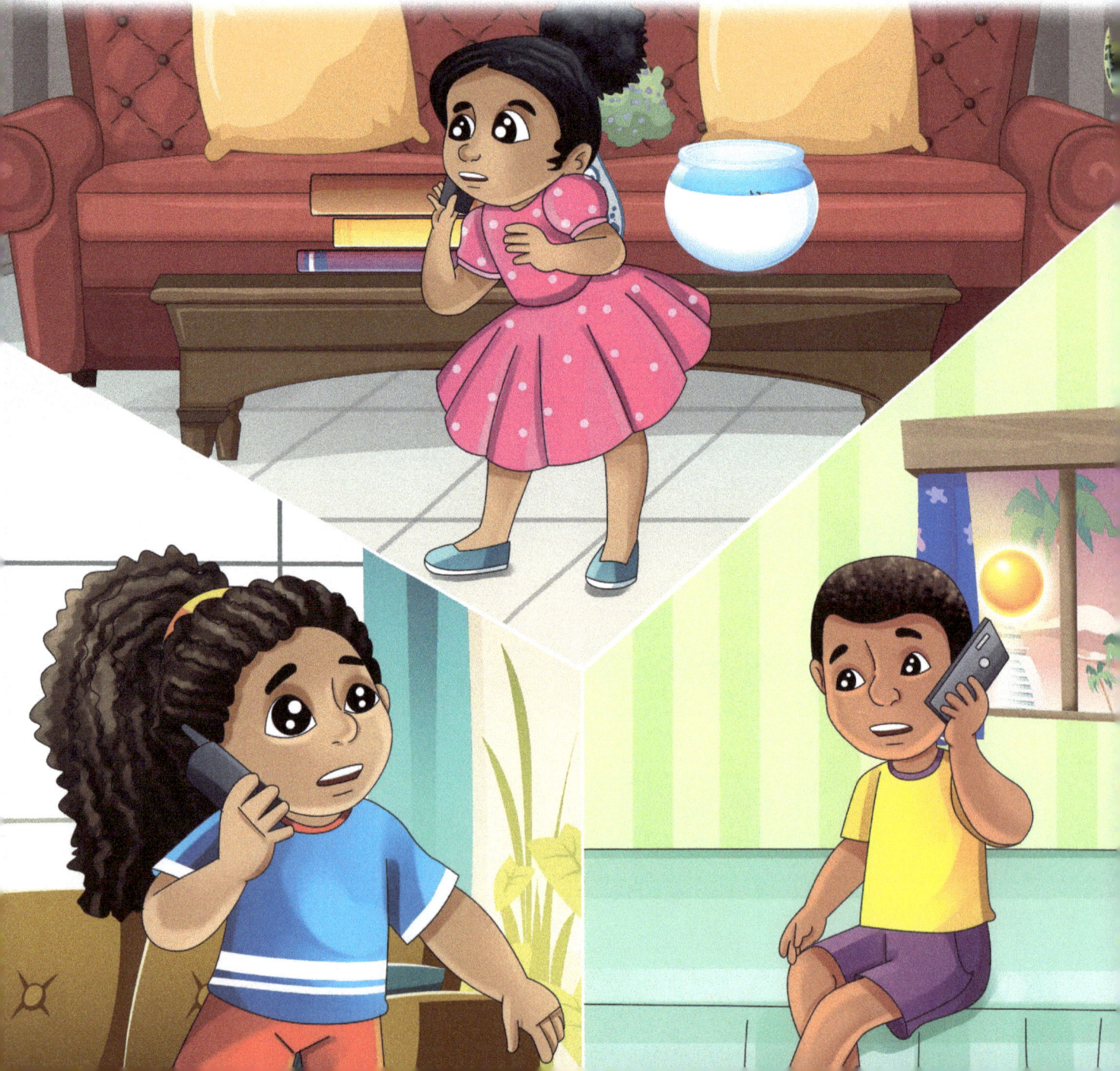

Corona there
Corona near,
Corona, you better leave this year!

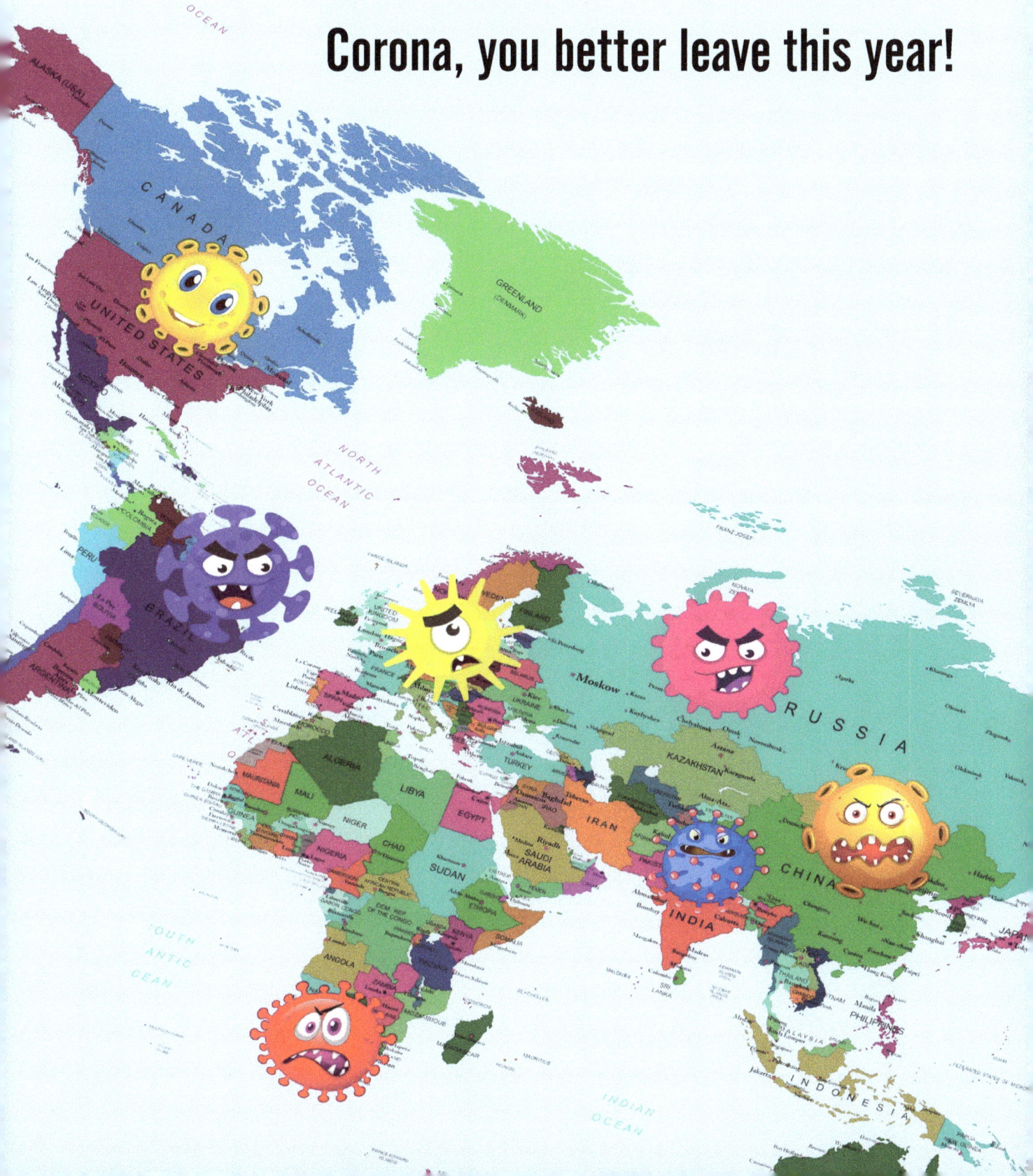

www.ingramcontent.com/pod-product-compliance
Lightning Source LLC
Chambersburg PA
CBHW041602260326
41914CB00011B/1362